KETO LUNCH RECIPES

KETO LUNCH RECIPES

58 Easy To Follow Recipes for Ketogenic Lunch

HEALTHY COOKING

COPYRIGHT ▌

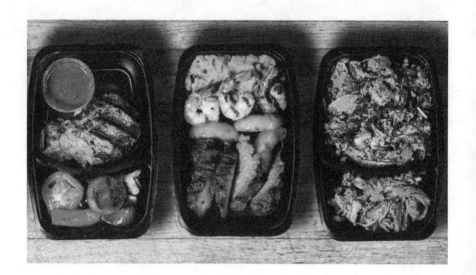

CONTENTS ▌

CONTENTS

CONTENTS

Introduction

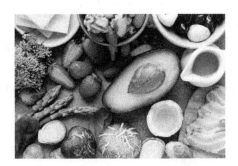

Even before we talk about how to do keto – it's important to first consider why this particular diet works. What actually happens to your body to make you lose weight?

As you probably know, the body uses food as an energy source. Everything you eat is turned into energy so that you can get up and do whatever you need to accomplish for the day. The main energy source is sugar so what happens is that you eat something, the body breaks it down into sugar, and the sugar is processed into energy. Typically, the "sugar" is taken directly from the food you eat so if you eat just the right amount of food, then your body is fueled for the whole day. If you eat too much, then the sugar is stored in your body – hence the accumulation of fat.

But what happens if you eat less food? This is where the Ketogenic Diet comes in. You see, the process of creating sugar from food is usually faster if the food happens to be rich in carbohydrates. Bread, rice, grain, pasta – all of these are carbohydrates and they're the easiest food types to turn into energy.

So the Ketogenic Diet is all about reducing the amount of carbohydrates you eat. Does this mean you won't get the kind of energy you need for the day? Of course not! It only means that now, your body has to find other possible sources of energy. Do you know where they will be getting that energy? Your stored body fat!

So here's the situation – you are eating less carbohydrates every day. To keep you energetic, the body breaks down the stored fat and turns them into molecules called ketone bodies. The process of turning the fat into ketone bodies is called "Ketosis" and obviously – this is where the name of the Ketogenic Diet comes from. The ketone bodies take the place of glucose in keeping you energetic. As long as you keep your carbohydrates reduced, the body will keep getting its energy from your body fat.

Sounds Simple, Right?

The Ketogenic Diet is often praised for its simplicity and when you look at it properly, the process is really straightforward. The Science behind the effectivity of the diet is also well-documented and has been proven multiple times by different medical fields. For example, an article on Diet Review by Harvard provided a lengthy discussion on how the Ketogenic Diet works and why it is so effective for those who choose to use this diet.

But Fat Is the Enemy...Or Is It?

No – fat is NOT the enemy. Unfortunately, years of bad science told us that fat is something you have to avoid – but it's actually a very helpful thing for weight loss! Even before we move forward with this book, we'll have to discuss exactly what "healthy fats" are, and why they're actually the good guys. To do this, we need to make a distinction between the different kinds of fat. You've probably heard of them before and it is a little bit confusing at first. We'll try to go through them as simply as possible:

Saturated fat. This is the kind you want to avoid. They're also called "solid fat" because each molecule is packed with hydrogen atoms. Simply put, it's the kind of fat that can easily cause a blockage in your body. It can raise cholesterol levels and lead to heart problems or a stroke. Saturated fat is something you can find in meat, dairy products, and other processed food items. Now, you're probably wondering: isn't the Ketogenic Diet packed with saturated fat? The answer is: not necessarily. You'll find later in the recipes given that the Ketogenic Diet promotes primarily unsaturated fat or healthy fat. While there are definitely many meat recipes in the list, most of these recipes contain healthy fat sources.

Unsaturated Fat. These are the ones dubbed as a healthy fat. They're the kind of fat you find in avocado, nuts, and other ingredients you usually find in Keto-friendly recipes. They're known to lower blood cholesterol and actually come in two types: polyunsaturated and monounsaturated. Both are good for your body but the benefits slightly vary, depending on what you're consuming.

Polyunsaturated fat. These are perhaps the best on the list. You know about omega-3 fatty acids right? They're often suggested for people who have heart problems and are recognized as the "healthy" kind of fat. Well, they fall under the category of polyunsaturated fat and are known for reducing risks of heart disease by as much as 19 percent. This is according to a study titled: Effects on coronary heart diseases of increased poly-unsaturated fat in lieu of saturated fat: systematic review & meta-analysis of randomized controlled tests. So where do you get these polyunsaturated fats? You can get them mostly from vegetable and seed oils. These are ingredients you can almost always find in Ketogenic Recipes such as olive oil, coconut oil, and more. If you need more convincing, you should also know that omega-3 fatty acids are actually a kind of polyunsaturated fats and you will find them in deep-sea fish like tuna, herring, and salmon.

What Is Keto And Why Is So Important For Your Health

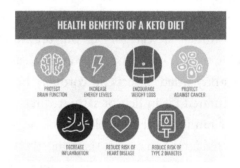

The health benefits of the Keto diet are not different for men or women, but the speed at which they are reached does differ. As mentioned, human bodies are a lot different when it comes to the ways that they are able to burn fats and lose weight. For example, by design women have at least 10% more body fat than men. No matter how fit you are, this is just an aspect of being a human that you must consider. Don't be hard on yourself if you notice that it seems like men can lose weight easier that's because they can! What women have in additional body fat, men typically have the same in muscle mass. This is why men tend to see faster external results, because that added muscle mass means that their metabolism rates are higher. That increased metabolism means that fat and energy get burned faster. When you are on Keto, though, the internal change is happening right away.

Your metabolism is unique, but it is also going to be slower than a man's by nature. Since muscle is able to burn more calories than fat, the weight just seems to fall off of men, giving them the ability to reach the opportunity for muscle growth quickly. This should not be something that holds you back from starting your Keto journey. As long as you are keeping these realistic bodily factors in mind, you won't be left wondering why it is taking you a little bit longer to start losing weight. This point will come for you, but it will take a little bit more of a process that you must be committed to following through with.

Another unique condition that a woman can experience but a man cannot be PCOS or Polycystic Ovary Syndrome; a hormonal imbalance that causes the development of cysts. These cysts can cause pain, interfere with normal reproductive function, and, in extreme and dangerous cases, burst. PCOS is actually very common among women, affecting up to 10% of the entire female population. Surprisingly, most women are not even aware that they have the condition. Around 70% of women have PCOS that is undiagnosed. This condition can cause a significant hormonal imbalance, therefore affecting your metabolism. It can also inevitably lead to weight gain, making it even harder to see results while following diet plans. In order to stay on top of your health, you must make sure that you are going to the gynecologist regularly.

Menopause is another reality that must be faced by women, especially as we age. Most women begin the process of menopause in their mid-40s. Men do not go through menopause, so they are spared from yet another condition that causes slower metabolism and weight gain. When you start menopause, it is easy to gain weight and lose muscle. Most women, once menopause begins, lose muscle at a much faster rate, and conversely gain weight, despite dieting and exercise regimens. Keto can, therefore, be the right diet plan for you. Regardless of what your body is doing naturally, via processes like menopause, your internal systems are still going to be making the switch from running on carbs to deriving energy from fats.

When the body begins to run on fats successfully, you have an automatic fuel reserving waiting to be burned. It will take some time for your body to do this, but when it does, you will actually be able to eat fewer calories and still feel just as full because your body knows to take energy from the fat that you already have. This will become automatic. It is, however, a process that requires some patience, but being aware of what is actually going on with your body can help you stay motivated while on Keto.

Because a Keto diet reduces the amount of sugar you are consuming, it naturally lowers the amount of insulin in your bloodstream. This can actually have amazing effects on any existing PCOS and fertility issues, as well as menopausal symptoms and conditions like pre-diabetes and Type 2 diabetes. Once your body adjusts to a Keto diet, you are overcoming the things that are naturally in place that can be preventing you from losing weight and getting healthy. Even if you placed your body on a strict diet, if it isn't getting rid of sugars properly, you likely aren't going to see the same results that you will when you try Keto. This is a big reason why Keto can be so beneficial for women.

You might not even realize that your hormones are not in balance until you experience a lifestyle that limits carbs and eliminates sugars. Keto is going to reset this balance for you, keeping your hormones at healthy levels. As a result of this, you will probably find yourself in a better general mood, and with much more energy to get through your days.

For people over 50, there are guidelines to follow when you start your Keto diet. As long as you are following the method properly and listening to what your body truly needs, you should have no more problems than men do while following the plan. What you will have are more obstacles to overcome, but you can do it. Remember that plenty of women successfully follow a Keto diet and see great results. Use these women as inspiration for how you anticipate your own journey to go. On the days when it seems impossible, remember what you have working against you, but more importantly what you have working for you. Your body is designed to go into ketogenesis more than it is designed to store fat by overeating carbs. Use this as a motivation to keep pushing you ahead. Keto is a valid option for you and the results will prove this, especially if you are over the age of 40.

Benefit of Keto Diet

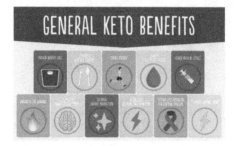

Benefits Ketogenic Diet

Reduction of cravings and appetite

Many people gain weight simply because they cannot control their cravings and appetite for caloric foods. The ketogenic diet helps eliminate these problems, but it does not mean that you will never be hungry or want to eat. You will feel hungry but only when you have to eat. Several studies have shown that the less carbohydrates you eat, the less you eat overall. Eating healthier foods that are high in fat helps reduce your appetite, as you lose more weight faster on a low-fat diet. The reason for this is that low carbohydrate diets help lower insulin levels, as your body does not need too much insulin to convert glycogen to glucose while eliminating excess water in your body. This diet helps you reduce visceral fat. In this way, you will get a slimmer look and shape. It is the most difficult fat to lose, as it surrounds the organs as it increases. High doses can cause inflammation and insulin resistance. Coconut oil can produce an immediate source of energy as it increases ketone levels in your body.

Reduction of risk of heart disease

Triglycerides, fat molecules in your body, have close links with heart disease. They are directly proportional as the more the number of triglycerides, the higher your chances of suffering from heart disease. You can reduce the number of free triglycerides in your body by reducing the number of carbohydrates, as is in the keto diets.

Reduces chances of having high blood pressure

Weight loss and blood pressure have a close connection; thus, since you are losing weight while on the keto diet, it will affect your blood pressure.

Fights type 2 diabetes

Type two diabetes develops as a result of insulin resistance. This is a result of having huge amounts of glucose in your system, with the keto diet this is not a possibility due to the low carbohydrate intake.

Increases the production of HDL

High-density lipoprotein is referred to as good cholesterol. It is responsible for caring calories to your liver, thus can be reused. High fat and low carbohydrate diets increase the production of HDL in your body, which also reduces your chances of getting a heart disease. Low-density lipoprotein is referred to as bad cholesterol.

Suppresses your appetite

It is a strange but true effect of the keto diet. It was thought that this was a result of the production of ketones but this was proven wrong as a study taken between people on a regular balanced diet and some on the keto diet and their appetites were generally the same. It, however, helps to suppress appetite as it is it has a higher fat content than many other diets. Food stays in the stomach for longer as fat and is digested slowly, thus provides a sense of fullness. On top of that, proteins promote the secretion cholecystokinin, which is a hormone that aids in regulating appetite. It is also believed that the ketogenic diet helps to suppress your appetite by continuous blunting of appetite. There is increased appetite in the initial stages of the diet, which decreases over time.

Changes in cholesterol levels

This is kind of on the fence between good and bad. This is because the ketogenic diet involves a high fat intake which makes people wonder about the effect on blood lipids and its potential to increase chances of heart disease and strokes, among others. Several major components play a lead role in determining this, which is: LDL, HDL, and blood triglyceride levels. Heart disease correlates with high levels of LDL and cholesterol. On the other hand, high levels of HDL are seen as protection from diseases caused by cholesterol levels. The impacts of the diet on cholesterol are not properly known. Some research has shown that there is no change in cholesterol levels while others have said that there is change. If you stay in deep ketosis for a very long period of time, your blood lipids will increase, but you will have to go through some negative effects of the ketogenic diet which will be corrected when the diet is over. If a person does not remain following the diet strictly for like ten years, he/she will not experience any cholesterol problems. It is difficult to differentiate the difference between diet and weight loss in general. The effect of the ketogenic diet on cholesterol has been boiled down to if you lose fat on the ketogenic diet then your cholesterol levels will go down, and if you don't lose fat, then your cholesterol levels will go up. Strangely, women have a larger cholesterol level addition than men, while both are on a diet. As there is no absolute conclusion on the effect of the ketogenic diet on cholesterol, you are advised to have your blood lipid levels constantly checked for any bad effects. Blood lipid levels should be checked before starting the diet and about eight weeks after starting. If repeated results show a worsening of lipid levels, then you should abandon the diet or substitute saturated fats with unsaturated fats.

Risk of a Ketogenic Diet

Low energy levels

When available, the body prefers to use carbohydrates for fuel as they burn more effectively than fats. General drop-in energy level is a concern raised by many dieters due to the lack of carbohydrates. Studies have shown that it causes orthostatic hypotension which causes lightheadedness. It has come to be known that these effects can be avoided by providing enough supplemental nutrients like sodium. Many of the symptoms can be prevented by providing 5 grams of sodium per day. Most times, fatigue disappears after a few weeks or even days, if fatigue doesn't disappear, then you should add a small number of carbohydrates to the diet as long as ketosis is maintained. The diet is not recommended when caring out high-intensity workouts, weight training, or high-intensity aerobic exercise as carbohydrates are an absolute requirement but are okay for low-intensity exercise.

Effects on the brain

It causes increased use of ketones by the brain. The increased use of ketones, among other reasons, result in the treating of childhood epilepsy. As a result of the changes that occur, the concern over the side effects, including permanent brain damage and short-term memory loss, has been raised. The origin of these concerns is difficult to understand. The brain is powered by ketones in the absence of glucose. Ketones are normal energy sources and not toxic as the brain creates enzymes, during fetal growth, that helps us use them. Epileptic children, though not the perfect examples, show some insight into the effects of the diet on the brain in the long term. There is no negative effect in terms of cognitive function. There is no assurance that the diet cannot have long term dietary effects, but no information proves that there are any negative effects. Some people feel they can concentrate more when on the ketogenic diet, while others feel nothing but fatigue. This is as a result of differences in individual physiology. There are very few studies that vaguely address the point on short term memory loss. This wore off with the continuation of the study.

Kidney stones and kidney damage

As a result of the increased workload from having to filter ketones, urea, and ammonia, as well as dehydration concerns of the potential for kidney damage or passing kidney stones have been raised. The high protein nature of the ketogenic diet raises the alarms of individuals who are concerned with potential kidney damage. There is very little information that points to any negative effects of the diet on kidney function or development of kidney stones. There is a low incidence of small kidney stones in epileptic children this may be as a result of the state of deliberate dehydration that the children are put at instead of the ketosis state itself. Some short term research shows no change in kidney function or increased incidents of kidney stones either after they are off the diet or after six months on a diet. There is no long term data on the effects of ketosis to kidney function; thus, no complete conclusions can be made. People with preexisting kidney issues are the only ones who get problems from high protein intake. From an unscientific point of view, one would expect increased incidents of this to happen to athletes who consume very high protein diets, but it has not happened. This suggests that high protein intake, under normal conditions, is not harmful to the kidneys. To limit the possibility of kidney stones, it is advised to drink a lot of water to maintain hydration. For people who are predisposed to kidney stones should have their kidney function should be monitored to ensure that no complications arise if they decide to follow through with the diet.

Constipation

A common side effect of the diet is reduced bowel movements and constipation. This arises from two different causes: lack of fiber and gastrointestinal absorption of foods. First, the lack of carbs in the diet means that unless supplements are taken, fiber intake is low. Fiber is very important to our systems. High fiber intake can prevent some health conditions, including heart disease and some forms of cancer. Use some type of sugar-free fiber supplement to prevent any health problems and help you maintain regular bowel movements. The diet also reduces the volume of stool due to enhanced absorption and digestion of food; thus, fewer waste products are generated.

Fat regain

Dieting, in general, has very low long term success rates. There are some effects of getting out of a ketogenic diet like the regain of fat lost through calorific restriction alone. This is true for any diet based on calorific restriction. It is expected for weight to be regained after carb reintroduction. For people who use the weighing scale to measure their success, they may completely shun carbs as they think it is the main reason for the weight regain. You should understand that most of the initial weight gain is water and glycogen.

Immune system

There is a large variety in the immunity system response to ketogenic diets on different people. There has been some repost on reduction on some ailments such allergies and increased minor sickness susceptibility.

Optic neuropathy

This is optic nerve dysfunction. It has appeared in a few cases, but it is still existence. It was linked to the people not getting adequate amounts of calcium or vitamins supplements for about a year. All the cases were corrected by supplementation of adequate vitamin B, especially thiamine.

4

Some Tips for Beginner to Achieve Keto Success

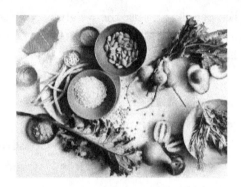

N

obody told you that life was going to be this way! But don't worry. There's still plenty of time to make amendments and take care of your health. Here are a couple of tips that will allow you to lead a healthier life in your fifties:

Start Building on Immunity

Every day, our body is exposed to free radicals and toxins from the environment. The added stress of work and family problems doesn't make it any easier for us. To combat this, it's essential that you start consuming healthy veggies that contain plenty of antioxidants and build a healthier immune system.

This helps ward off unwanted illnesses and diseases, allowing you to maintain good health.

Adding more healthy veggies to your Keto diet will help you obtain a variety of minerals, vitamins and antioxidants.

Consider Quitting Smoking

It's never too late to try to quit smoking even if you are in your fifties. Once a smoker begins to quit, the body quickly starts to heal the previous damages caused by smoking.

Once you start quitting, you'll notice how you'll be able to breathe easier, while acquiring a better sense of smell and taste. Over the period of time, eliminating the habit of smoking can greatly reduce the risks of high blood pressure, strokes and heart attack. Please note how these diseases are much more common among folks who are in the fifties and above when compared to younger folks.

Not to mention, quitting smoking will help you stay more active and enjoy better health with your friends and family.

Stay Social

We've already mentioned this before but it's worth pondering on again and again. Aging can be a daunting process and trying to get through it all on your own isn't particularly helpful. We urge you to stay in touch with friends and family or become a part of a local community club or network. Some older folks find it comforting to get an emotional support animal.

Being surrounded by people you love will give you a sense of belonging and will improve your mood. It'll also keep your mind and memory sharp as you engage in different conversations.

Health Screenings You Should Get After Your Fifties

Your fifties are considered the prime years of your life. Don't let the joy of these years be robbed away from you because of poor health. Getting simple tests done can go a long way in identifying any potential health problems that you may have. Here is a list of health screenings should get done:

Check Your Blood Pressure

Your blood pressure is a reliable indicator of your heart health. In simple words, blood pressure is a measure of how fast blood travels through the artery walls. Very high or even very low blood pressure can be a sign of an underlying problem. Once you hit your 40s, you should have your blood pressure checked more often.

EKG

The EKG reveals your heart health and activity. Short for electro-cardiogram, the EKG helps identify problems in the heart. The process works by highlighting any rhythm problems that may be in the heart such as poor heart muscles, improper blood flow or any other form of abnormality. Getting an EKG is also a predictive measure for understanding the chances of a heart attack. Since people starting their fifties are at greater risk of getting a heart attack, you should get yourself checked more often.

Mammogram

Mammograms help rule out the risks of breast cancer. Women who enter their fifties should ideally get a mammogram after every ten years. However, if you have a family history, it is advisable that you get one much earlier to rule out the possibilities of cancer.

Blood Sugar Levels

If you're somebody who used to grab a fast food meal every once in a while before you switched to Keto, then you should definitely check your blood sugar levels more carefully. Blood sugar levels indicate whether or not you have diabetes. And you know how the saying goes, prevention is better than cure. It's best to clear these possibilities out of the way sooner than later.

Check for Osteoporosis

Unfortunately, as you grow older you also become susceptible to a number of bone diseases. Osteoporosis is a bone-related condition in which bones begin to lose mass, becoming frail and weak. Owing to this, seniors become more prone to fractures. This can make even the smallest of falls detrimental to your health.

Annual Physical Exam

Your insurance must be providing coverage for your annual physical exam. So, there's no reason you should not take advantage of it. This checkup helps identify the state of your health. You'll probably be surprised by how much doctors can tell from a single blood test.

Prostrate Screening Exam

Once men hit their fifties, they should be screened for prostate cancer (similar to how women should get a mammogram and pap smear). Getting a screening done becomes especially important if cancer runs in your family.

Eye Exam

As you start to age, you'll notice how your eyesight will start to deteriorate. It's quite likely that vision is not as sharp as it used to be. Ideally, you should have gotten your first eye exam during your 40s but it isn't too late. Get one as soon as possible to prevent symptoms from escalating.

Be Wary of Any Weird Moles

While skin cancer can become a problem at any age, older adults should pay closer attention to any moles or unusual skin tags in their bodies. While most cancers can be easily treated, melanoma can be particularly quite dangerous. If you have noticed any recent moles in your body that have changed in color, size or shape, make sure to visit the dermatologist.

Check Your Cholesterol Levels

Now, we've talked about this plenty of times but it's worth mentioning again. High cholesterol levels can be dangerous to your health and can be an indicator for a number of diseases, things become more complicated for conditions that don't show particular symptoms. Just to be on the safe side, your total cholesterol levels should be below 200 mg per deciliter. Your doctor will take a simple blood test and will give you a couple of guidelines with the results. In case there is something to worry about, you should make serious dietary and lifestyle changes in your life.

5

What does the ketogenic diet mean to women?

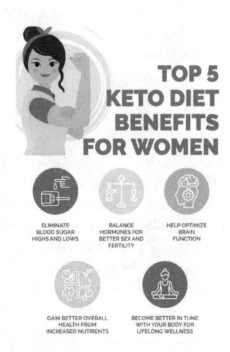

Why Keto for Women?

The health benefits of the Keto diet are not different for men or women, but the speed at which they are reached does differ. As mentioned, women's bodies are a lot different when it comes to the ways that they are able to burn fats and lose weight. For example, by design women have at least 10% more body fat than men. No matter how fit you are, this is just an aspect of being a woman that you must consider. Don't be hard on yourself if you notice that it seems like men can lose weight easier — that's because they can! What women have in additional body fat; men typically have the same in muscle mass. This is why men tend to see faster external results, because that added muscle mass means that their metabolism rates are higher. That increased metabolism means that fat and energy get burned faster. When you are on Keto, though, the internal change is happening right away.

Your metabolism is unique, but it is also going to be slower than a man's by nature. Since muscle is able to burn more calories than fat, the weight just seems to fall off of men, giving them the ability to reach the opportunity for muscle growth quickly. This should not be something that holds you back from starting your Keto journey. As long as you are keeping these realistic bodily factors in mind, you won't be left wondering why it is taking you a little bit longer to start losing weight. This point will come for you, but it will take a little bit more of a process that you must be committed to following through with.

Another unique condition that a woman can experience but a man cannot be PCOS or Polycystic Ovary Syndrome; a hormonal imbalance that causes the development of cysts. These cysts can cause pain, interfere with normal reproductive function, and, in extreme and dangerous cases, burst. PCOS is actually very common among women, affecting up to 10% of the entire female population. Surprisingly, most women are not even aware that they have the condition. Around 70% of women have PCOS that is undiagnosed. This condition can cause a significant hormonal imbalance, therefore affecting your metabolism. It can also inevitably lead to weight gain, making it even harder to see results while following diet plans. In order to stay on top of your health, you must make sure that you are going to the gynecologist regularly.

Menopause is another reality that must be faced by women, especially as we age. Most women begin the process of menopause in their mid-40s. Men do not go through menopause, so they are spared from yet another condition that causes slower metabolism and weight gain. When you start menopause, it is easy to gain weight and lose muscle. Most women, once menopause begins, lose muscle at a much faster rate, and conversely gain weight, despite dieting and exercise regimens. Keto can, therefore, be the right diet plan for you. Regardless of what your body is doing naturally, via processes like menopause, your internal systems are still going to be making the switch from running on carbs to deriving energy from fats.

Because a Keto diet reduces the amount of sugar you are consuming, it naturally lowers the amount of insulin in your bloodstream. This can actually have amazing effects on any existing PCOS and fertility issues, as well as menopausal symptoms and conditions like pre-diabetes and Type 2 diabetes. Once your body adjusts to a Keto diet, you are overcoming the things that are naturally in place that can be preventing you from losing weight and getting healthy. Even if you placed your body on a strict diet, if it isn't getting rid of sugars properly, you likely aren't going to see the same results that you will when you try Keto. This is a big reason why Keto can be so beneficial for women.

As we've deliberated, carbs and sugar can have a huge impact on your hormonal balance. You might not even realize that your hormones are not in balance until you experience a lifestyle that limits carbs and eliminates sugars. Keto is going to reset this balance for you, keeping your hormones at healthy levels. As a result of this, you will probably find yourself in a better general mood, and with much more energy to get through your days.

Why Keto for 40+?

As we age, we naturally look for ways to hold onto our youth and energy. It's not uncommon to think about things that promote anti-aging. Products and lifestyle changes are advertised everywhere, and they are designed to catch your attention, as you grapple with the reality of what it means to be a 40+ year-old woman in our society. Even if you aren't eating for the purposes of anti-aging yet, you have likely thought about it in terms of the way you treat your skin and hair, for example. The great thing about the Keto diet is that it supports maximum health, from the inside out; working hard to make sure that you are in the best shape that you can be in.

For instance, indigestion becomes common as you age. This happens because the body is not able to break down certain foods as well as it used to. With all of the additives and fillers, we all become used to putting our bodies through discomfort in an attempt to digest regular meals. You are probably not even aware that you are doing this to your body, but upon trying a Keto diet, you will realize how your digestion will begin to change. You will no longer feel bloated or uncomfortable after you eat. If you notice this as a common feeling, you are likely not eating food that is nutritious enough to satisfy your needs and is only resulting in excess calories.

Keto fills you up in all of the ways that you need, allowing your body to truly digest and metabolize all of the nutrients. When you eat your meals, you should not feel the need to overeat in order to overcompensate for not having enough nutrients. Anything that takes stress off of any system in your body is going to become a form of anti-aging. You will quickly find this benefit once you start your Keto journey, as it is one of the first-reported changes that most participants notice. In addition to a healthier digestive system, you will also experience more regular bathroom usage, with little to none of the problems often associated with age.

While weight loss is one of the more common desires for most 40+ women who start a diet plan, the way that the weight is lost matters. If you have ever shed a lot of weight before, you have probably experienced the adverse effects of sagging or drooping skin that you were left to deal with. Keto actually rejuvenates the elasticity in your skin. This means that you will be able to lose weight and your skin will be able to catch up. Instead of having to do copious amounts of exercise to firm up your skin, it should already be becoming firmer each day that you are on the Keto diet. This is something that a lot of participants are pleasantly surprised to find out.

Women also commonly report a natural reduction in wrinkles, and healthier skin and hair growth, in general. Many women who start the diet report that they actually notice reverse effects in their aging process. While the skin becomes healthier and more supple, it also becomes firmer. Even if you aren't presently losing weight, you will still be able to appreciate the effects that Keto brings to your skin and face. Because your internal systems are becoming healthier by the day, this tends to show on the outside in a short amount of time. You will also begin to feel healthier. While it is possible to read about the experiences of others, there is nothing like feeling this for yourself when you begin Keto.

Everyone, especially women over 40, has day-to-day tasks that are draining and require certain amounts of energy to complete. Aging can, unfortunately, take away from your energy reserve, even if you get enough sleep at night. It limits the way that you have to live your life, and this can become a very frustrating realization. Most diet plans bring about a sluggish feeling that you are simply supposed to get used to, for example. But Keto does the exact opposite. When you change your eating habits to fit the Keto guidelines, you are going to be hit with a boost of energy. Since your body is truly getting everything that it needs nutritionally, it will repay you with a sustained energy supply.

Another common complaint for women over 40 is that, seemingly overnight, your blood sugar levels are going to be more sensitive than usual. While it is important that everyone keeps an eye on these levels, it is especially important for those who are in their 50s and beyond. High blood sugar can be an indication that diabetes is on the way, but Keto can become a preventative measure, that we've already talked about. Additionally, naturally regulating elevated blood sugar levels, also reduces systemic inflammation, which is also common for women over 50. By balancing the immune system, of which inflammation is a part of, common aches and pains are reduced. Inflammation can also affect vital organs and is a precursor to cancer. Keto will support your path to an anti-inflammatory lifestyle.

Sugar is never great for us, but it turns out that sugar can become especially dangerous as we age. What is known as a "sugar sag" can occur when you get older because the excess sugar molecules will attach themselves to skin and protein in your body. This doesn't even necessarily happen because you are eating too much sugar. Average levels of sugar intake can also lead to this sagging as the sugar weakens the strength of your proteins that are supposed to hold you together. With sagging comes even more wrinkles and arterial stiffening.

If you have any anti-aging concerns, the Keto diet will likely be able to address your worries. It is a diet that works extremely hard while allowing you a fairly simple and direct guideline to follow in return. While your motivation is necessary in order to form a successful relationship with Keto, you won't need to worry about doing anything "wrong" or accidentally breaking from your diet. As long as you know how to give up your sugary foods and drinks while making sure that you are consuming the correct amount of carbs, you will be able to find your own success while on the diet.

As a woman over 50, you'll find that you will feel better, healthier and younger, by implementing the simple steps that will tune your body into processing excess fats for energy. You'll build muscle, lose fat, and look and feel younger. As we've touched on, a Keto diet helps balance your hormones, reversing and/or eliminating many common menopausal signs and symptoms.

6

What Keto Does to a Woman's Body

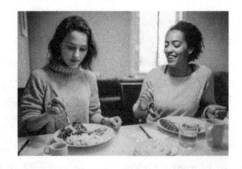

Women who are looking for a quick and effective way to shed excess weight, get high blood sugar levels under control, reduce overall inflammations, and improve physical and mental energy will do their best by following a ketogenic diet plan. But there are special considerations women must take into account when they are beginning the keto diet.

All women know it is much more difficult for women to lose weight than it is for men to lose weight. A woman will live on a starvation level diet and exercise like a triathlete and only lose five pounds. A man will stop putting dressing on his salad and will lose twenty pounds. It just is not fair. But we have the fact that we are women to blame. Women naturally have more standing between them and weight loss than men do.

The mere fact that we are women is the largest single contributor to the reason we find it difficult to lose weight. Since our bodies always think they need to be prepared for the possibility of pregnancy women will naturally have more body fat and less mass in our muscles than men will. Muscle cells burn more calories than fat cells do. So, because we are women, we will always lose weight more slowly than men will.

Being in menopause will also cause women to add more pounds to their bodies, especially in the lower half of the body. After menopause a woman's metabolism naturally slows down. Your hormones levels will decrease. These two factors alone will cause weight gain in the post-menopausal woman.

Women are a direct product of their hormones. Men also have hormones but not the ones like we have that regulate every function in our bodies. And the hormones in women will fluctuate around their everyday habits like lack of sleep, poor eating habits, and menstrual cycles. These hormones cause women to crave sweets around the time their periods occur. These cravings will wreck any diet plan. Staying true to the keto plan is challenging at this time because of the intense craving for sweets and carbs. Also having your period will often make you feel and look bloated because of the water your body holds onto during this time. And having cramps make you more likely to reach for a bag of cookies than a plate of steak and salad.

Because we are women, we may experience challenges on the keto diet that men will not face because they are men. One of these challenges is having weight loss plateau or even experiencing weight gain. This can happen because of the influence of hormones on weight loss in women. If this happens you will want to increase your consumption of good fats like ghee, butter, eggs, coconut oil, beef, avocados, and olive oil. Any food that is cooked or prepared using oil must be prepared in olive oil or avocado oil.

You can also use MCT oil. MCT stands for medium chain triglycerides. This is a form of fatty acid that is saturated and has many health benefits. MCT can help with many body functions from weight loss to improved brain function. MCTs are mostly missing from the typical American diet because we have been told that saturated fats are harmful to the body, and as a group they are. But certain saturated fats, like MCTs, are actually beneficial to the body, especially when they come from good foods like beef or coconut oil. They are easier to digest than most other saturated fats and may help improve heart and brain function and prevent obesity.

Many women on a keto diet will struggle with imbalances in their hormones. On the keto diet you do not rely on lowered calories to lose weight but on foods effect on your hormones. So, when women begin the keto diet any issues, they are already having with their hormones will be brought to attention and may cause the woman to give up before she really begins. Always remember that the keto diet is responsible for cleansing the system first so that the body can easily respond to the wonderful affects a keto diet has to offer.

Do not try to work toward the lean body that many men sport. It is best for overall function that women stay at twenty-two to twenty six percent body fat. Our hormones will function best in this range and we can't possibly function without our hormones. Women who are very lean, like gymnasts and extreme athletes, will find their hormones no longer function or function at a less than optimal rate. And remember that ideal weight may not be the right weight for you. Many women find that they perform their best when they are at their happy weight. If you find yourself fighting with yourself to lose the last few pounds you think you need to lose in order to have the perfect body then it may not be worth it. The struggle will affect your hormone function. Carefully observing the keto diet will allow time for your hormones to stabilize and regulate themselves back to their pre-obesity normal function.

Like any other diet plan the keto diet will work better if you are active. Regular exercise will allow the body to strengthen and tone muscles and will help to work off excess fat reserves. But exercise requires energy to accomplish. If you restrict your carb intake too much you might not have the energy needed to be physically able to make it all the way through the day and still be able to maintain an exercise routine. You might need to add in more carbs to your diet through the practice of carb cycling.

As a woman you know that sometimes your emotions get the better of you. This is true with your body, as you well know, and can be a major reason why women find it extremely difficult at times to lose weight the way they want to lose weight. We have been led to believe that not only can we do it all but that we must do it all. This gives many women unnecessary levels of pressure and can cause them to engage in emotional eating. Some women might have lowered feelings of self-worth and may not feel they are entitled to the benefits of the keto diet, and turning to food relieves the feelings of inadequacy that we try to hide from the world.

When you engage in the same activity for a long period of time it becomes a habit. When you reach for the bag of potato chips or the tub of ice cream whenever you are angry, upset, or depressed, then your brain will eventually tell you to reach for food whenever you feel an emotion that you don't want to deal with. Food acts as a security blanket against the world outside. It may be necessary to address any extreme emotional issues you are having before you begin the keto diet, so that you are better assured of success.

The basic act of staying on the keto diet can be very challenging for some women. Many women see beginning a new diet to lose weight as a punishment for being overweight. It may be worthwhile for you to work at changing the set of your mind if you are feeling this way. You may need to remind yourself daily that the keto diet is not a punishment but a blessing for your body. Tell yourself that you are not denying yourself certain foods because you can't eat them, but because you do not like the way those foods make your body feel. Don't watch other people eating their high carb diet and pity yourself. Instead, feel sorry for the people who have trapped themselves in a high calorie diet and are not experiencing the benefits that you are experiencing.

And for the first thirty days cut out all sweeteners, even the non-sugar ones that are allowed on the keto diet. While they may make food taste better, they also remind your brain that it needs sweet foods when it really doesn't. Cutting them out for at least thirty days will break the cycle that your body has fallen into and will cut the cravings for sweets in your diet.

It is very possible for women to be successful on the keto diet if they are prepared to follow a few simple adjustments that will make the diet look differently than your male partner might be eating but that will make you successful in the long run.

During the first one or two weeks you will need to consume extra fat than a man might need to. Doing this will have three important effects on your body. First it will cause your mitochondria to intensify their acceptance of your new way of finding energy. Mitochondria are tiny organisms that are found in cells and are responsible for using the fuel that insulin brings to the cell for fuel for the cell. Increasing your fat intake will also help make sure you are getting enough calories in your daily diet. This is important because if your body thinks you are starving it will begin to conserve calories and you will stop losing weight.

The third benefit from eating more fat, and perhaps the most important, is the psychological boost you will get from seeing that you can eat more fat and still lose weight and feel good. It will also reset your mindset that you formerly might have held against fat. For so long we have been told that low fat is the only way to lose weight. But an absence of dietary fat will lead to overeating and binge eating out of a feeling of deprivation. When you begin the diet by allowing yourself to eat a lot, or too much in your mind, fat, then you swing the pendulum around to the other side of the fat scale where it properly belongs. You teach yourself that fat can be good for you. Increasing the extra intake of fats should not last beyond the second week of the diet. Your body will improve its abilities to create and burn ketones and body fat, and then you will begin using your own body fat for fuel and you can begin to lower your reliance on dietary fat a little bit so that you will begin to lose weight.

The keto diet is naturally lower in calories if you follow the recommended levels of food intake. It is not necessary to try to restrict your intake of calories even further. All you need to do is to eat only until you are full and not one bite more. Besides losing weight the aim of the keto diet is to retrain your body on how to work properly. You will need to learn to trust your body and the signals it sends out to be able to readjust to a proper way of eating.

7

How Can Ketogenic Diet Can Aid With the Sign and Symptoms of Ageing and Menopause

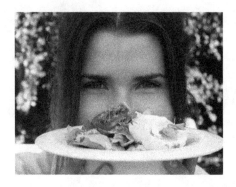

How the ketogenic diet can aid with the signs and symptoms of ageing and menopause

For ageing women, menopause will bring severe changes and challenges, but the ketogenic diet can help you switch gears effortlessly to continue enjoying a healthy and happy life. Menopause can upset hormonal levels in women, which consequently affects brainpower and cognitive abilities. Furthermore, due to less production of estrogens and progesterone, your sex drive declines, and you suffer from sleep issues and mood problems. Let's have a look at how a ketogenic diet will help solve these side effects.

Enhanced Cognitive Functions

Usually, hormone estrogen ensures continuous flow of glucose into your brain. But after menopause, the estrogen levels begin to drop dramatically, so does the amount of glucose reaching the bran. As a result, your functional brainpower will start to deteriorate. However, by following the keto diet for women over 50, the problem of glucose intake is circumvented. This results in enhanced cognitive functions and brain activity.

Hormonal Balance

Usually, women face major symptoms of menopause due to hormonal imbalances. The keto diet for women over 50 works by stabilizing these imbalances such as estrogen. This aids in experiencing fewer and bearable menopausal symptoms like hot flashes. The keto diet also balances blood sugar levels and insulin and helps in controlling insulin sensitivity.

Intensified Sex Drive

The keto diet surges the absorption of vitamin D, which is essential for enhancing sex drive. Vitamin D ensures stable levels of testosterone and other sex hormones that could become unstable due to low levels of testosterone.

Better Sleep

Glucose disturbs your blood sugar levels dramatically, which in turn leads to poor quality of sleep. Along with other menopausal symptoms, good sleep becomes a huge problem as you age. The keto diet for women over 50 not only balances blood glucose levels, but also stabilizes other hormones like cortisol, melatonin, and serotonin warranting an improved and better sleep.

Reduces inflammation

Menopause can upsurge the inflammation levels by letting potential harmful invaders in our system, which result in uncomfortable and painful symptoms. Keto diet for women over 50 uses the healthy anti-inflammatory fats to reduce inflammation and lower pain in your joints and bones.

Fuel your brain

Are you aware that your brain is composed of 60% fat or more? This infers that it needs a larger amount of fat to keep it functioning optimally. In other words, the ketones from the keto diet serve as the energy source that fuels your brain cells.

Nutrient deficiencies

Ageing women tend to have higher deficiencies in essential nutrients such as, iron deficiency which leads to brain fog and fatigue; Vitamin B12 deficiency, which lead to neurological conditions like dementia; Fats deficiency, that can lead to problems with cognition, skin, vision; and Vitamin D deficiency that not only causes cognitive impairment in older adults and increase the risk of heart disease but also contribute to the risk of developing cancer. On a keto diet, the high-quality proteins ensure adequate and excellent sources of these important nutrients.

Controlling Blood Sugar

Research has suggested a link between poor blood sugar levels and brain diseases such as Alzheimer's disease, Parkinson's disease, or Dementia. Some factors contributing to Alzheimer's disease may include:

- Enormous intake of carbohydrates, especially from fructose—which is drastically reduced in the ketogenic diet.

- Lack of nutritional fats and good cholesterol — which are copious and healthy in the keto diet

Keto diet helps control blood sugar and improve nutrition; which in turn not only improve insulin response and resistance but also protect against memory loss which is often a part of ageing.

8

Foods Allowed in Keto Diet

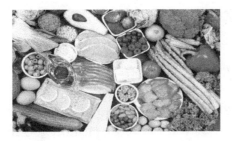

To make the most of your diet, there are prohibited foods, and others that are allowed, but in limited quantities. Here are the foods allowed in the ketogenic diet:

Food allowed in unlimited quantities

Lean or fatty meats

No matter which meat you choose, it contains no carbohydrates so that you can have fun! Pay attention to the quality of your meat, and the amount of fat. Alternate between fatty meats and lean meats!

Here are some examples of lean meats:

Beef: sirloin steak, roast beef, 5% minced steak, roast, flank steak, tenderloin, Grisons meat, tripe, kidneys

Horse: roti, steak

Pork: tenderloin, bacon, kidneys

Veal: cutlet, shank, tenderloin, sweetbread, liver

Chicken and turkey: cutlet, skinless thigh, ham

Rabbit

Here are some examples of fatty meats:

Lamb: leg, ribs, brain

Beef: minced steak 10, 15, 20%, ribs, rib steak, tongue, marrow

Pork: ribs, brain, dry ham, black pudding, white pudding, bacon, terrine, rillettes, salami, sausage, sausages, and merguez

Veal: roast, paupiette, marrow, brain, tongue, dumplings

Chicken and turkey: thigh with skin

Guinea fowl

Capon

Turkey

Goose: foie gras

Lean or fatty fish

The fish does not contain carbohydrates so that you can consume unlimited! As with meat, there are lean fish and fatty fish, pay attention to the amount of fat you eat and remember to vary your intake of fish. Oily fish have the advantage of containing a lot of good cholesterol, so it is beneficial for protection against cardiovascular disease! It will be advisable to consume fatty fish more than lean fish, to be able to manage your protein intake: if you consume lean fish, you will have a significant protein intake and little lipids, whereas with fatty fish, you will have a balanced protein and fat intake!

Here are some examples of lean fish:

- Cod
- Colin
- Sea bream
- Whiting
- Sole
- Turbot
- Limor career

- Location
- Pike
- Ray

Here are some examples of oily fish:

- Swordfish
- Salmon
- Tuna
- Trout
- Monkfish
- Herring
- Mackerel
- Cod
- Sardine

Eggs

The eggs contain no carbohydrates, so you can consume as much as you want. It is often said that eggs are full of cholesterol and that you have to limit their intake, but the more cholesterol you eat, the less your body will produce by itself! In addition, it's not just poor-quality cholesterol so that you can consume 6 per week without risk! And if you want to eat more but you are afraid for your cholesterol and I have not convinced you, remove the yellow!

Vegetables and raw vegetables

Yes, you can eat vegetables. But you have to be careful which ones: you can eat leafy vegetables (salad, spinach, kale, red cabbage, Chinese cabbage...) and flower vegetables (cauliflower, broccoli, Romanesco cabbage...) as well as avocado, cucumbers, zucchini or leeks, which do not contain many carbohydrates.

The oils

It's oil, so it's only fat, so it's unlimited to eat, but choose your oil wisely! Prefer olive oil, rapeseed, nuts, sunflower or sesame for example!

Foods authorized in moderate quantities.

The cold cuts

As you know, there is bad cholesterol in cold meats, so you will need to moderate your intake: eat it occasionally!

Fresh cheeses and plain yogurts

Consume with moderation because they contain carbohydrates.

Nuts and oilseeds

They have low levels of carbohydrates, but are rich in saturated fatty acids, that's why they should moderate their consumption. Choose almonds, hazelnuts, Brazil nuts or pecans.

Coconut (in oil, cream or milk)

It contains saturated fatty acids, that's why we limit its consumption. Cream and coconut oil contain a lot of medium chain triglycerides (MCTs), which increase the level of ketones, essential to stay in ketosis.

Berries and red fruits

They contain carbohydrates, in reasonable quantities, but you should not abuse them to avoid ketosis (blueberries, blackberries, raspberries...).

9

Keto Grocery List

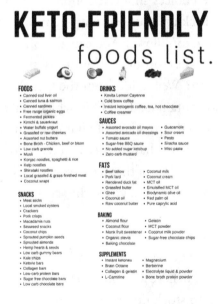

KETO-FRIENDLY
foods list.

FOODS
- Canned cod liver oil
- Canned tuna & salmon
- Canned sardines
- Free range organic eggs
- Fermented pickles
- Kimchi & sauerkraut
- Water buffalo yogurt
- Grassfed or raw cheeses
- Assorted nut butters
- Bone Broth - Chicken, beef or bison
- Low carb granola
- Musli
- Konjac noodles, spaghetti & rice
- Kelp noodles
- Shirataki noodles
- Local grassfed & grass finished meat
- Coconut wraps

SNACKS
- Meat sticks
- Local smoked oysters
- Crackers
- Pork crisps
- Macadamia nuts
- Seaweed snacks
- Coconut chips
- Sprouted pumpkin seeds
- Sprouted almonds
- Hemp hearts & seeds
- Low carb gummy bears
- Kale chips
- Ketone bars
- Collagen bars
- Low-carb protein bars
- Sugar free chocolate bars
- Low carb chocolate bars

DRINKS
- Kevita Lemon Cayenne
- Cold brew coffee
- Instant ketogenic coffee, tea, hot chocolate
- Coffee creamer

SAUCES
- Assorted avocado oil mayos
- Assorted avocado oil dressings
- Tomato sauce
- Sugar-free BBQ sauce
- No added sugar ketchup
- Zero carb mustard
- Guacamole
- Sour cream
- Pesto
- Siracha sauce
- Miso paste

FATS
- Beef tallow
- Pork lard
- Rendered duck fat
- Grassfed butter
- Ghee
- Coconut oil
- Raw coconut butter
- Coconut milk
- Coconut cream
- MCT oil
- Emulsified MCT oil
- Biodynamic olive oil
- Red palm oil
- Pure caprylic acid

BAKING
- Almond flour
- Coconut flour
- Monk fruit sweetener
- Organic stevia
- Baking chocolate
- Gelatin
- MCT powder
- Coconut milk powder
- Sugar-free chocolate chips

SUPPLEMENTS
- Instant ketones
- Brain Octane
- Collagen & gelatin
- L-Carnitine
- Magnesium
- Berberine
- Electrolyte liquid & powder
- Bone broth protein powder

I've had people complain about the difficulty of switching their grocery list to one that's Ketogenic-friendly. The fact is that food is expensive – and most of the food you have in your fridge are probably packed full with carbohydrates. This is why if you're committing to a Ketogenic Diet, you need to do a clean sweep. That's right – everything that's packed with carbohydrates should be identified and set aside to make sure you're not eating more than you should. You can donate them to a charity before going out and buying your new Keto-friendly shopping list.

Seafood

Seafood means fish like sardines, mackerel, and wild salmon. It's also a good idea to add some shrimp, tuna, mussels, and crab into your diet. This is going to be a tad expensive but definitely worth it in the long run. What's the common denominator in all these food items? The secret is omega-3 fatty acids which is credited for lots of health benefits. You want to add food rich in omega-3 fatty acids in your diet.

Low-carb Vegetables

Not all vegetables are good for you when it comes to the Ketogenic Diet. The vegetable choices should be limited to those with low carbohydrate counts. Pack up your cart with items like spinach, eggplant, arugula, broccoli, and cauliflower. You can also put in bell peppers, cabbage, celery, kale, Brussels sprouts, mushrooms, zucchini, and fennel.

So what's in them? Well, aside from the fact that they're low-carb, these vegetable also contain loads of fiber which makes digestion easier. Of course, there's also the presence of vitamins, minerals, antioxidants, and various other nutrients that you need for day to day life. Which ones should you avoid? Steer clear of the starch-packed vegetables like carrots, turnips, and beets. As a rule, you go for the vegetables that are green and leafy.

Fruits Low in Sugar

During an episode of sugar-craving, it's usually a good idea to pick low-sugar fruit items. Believe it or not, there are lots of those in the market! Just make sure to stock up on any of these: avocado, blackberries, raspberries, strawberries, blueberries, lime, lemon, and coconut. Also note that tomatoes are fruits too so feel free to make side dishes or dips with loads of tomatoes! Keep in mind that these fruits should be eaten fresh and not out of a can. If you do eat them fresh off the can however, take a good look at the nutritional information at the back of the packaging. Avocadoes are particularly popular for those practicing the Ketogenic Diet because they contains LOTS of the good kind of fat.

Meat and Eggs

While some diets will tell you to skip the meat, the Ketogenic Diet actually encourages its consumption. Meat is packed with protein that will feed your muscles and give you a consistent source of energy through the day. It's a slow but sure burn when you eat protein as opposed to carbohydrates which are burned faster and therefore stored faster if you don't use them immediately.

But what kind of meat should you be eating? There's chicken, beef, pork, venison, turkey, and lamb. Keep in mind that quality plays a huge role here – you should be eating grass-fed organic beef or organic poultry if you want to make the most out of this food variety. The organic option lets you limit the possibility of ingesting toxins in your body due to the production process of these products. Plus, the preservation process also means there are added salt or sugar in the meat, which can throw off the whole diet.

Nuts and Seeds

Nuts and seeds you should definitely add in your cart include: chia seeds, Brazil nuts, macadamia nuts, flaxseed, walnuts, hemp seeds, pecans, sesame seeds, almonds, hazelnut, and pumpkin seeds. They also contain lots of protein and very little sugar so they're great if you have the munchies. They're the ideal snack because they're quick, easy, and will keep you full. They're high in calories though, which is why lots of people steer clear of them. As I mentioned earlier though – the Ketogenic Diet has nothing to do with calories and everything to do with the nutrient you're eating. So don't pay too much attention on the calorie count and just remember that they're a good source of fats and protein.

Dairy Products

OK – some people in their 50s already have a hard time processing dairy products, but for those who don't – you can happily add many of these to your diet. Make sure to consume sufficient amounts of cheese, plain Greek yogurt, cream butter, and cottage cheese. These dairy products are packed with calcium, protein, and the healthy kind of fat.

Oils

Nope, we're not talking about essentials oils but rather, MCT oil, coconut oil, avocado oil, nut oils, and even extra-virgin olive oil. You can start using those for your frying needs to create healthier food options. The beauty of these oils is that they add flavor to the food, making sure you don't get bored quickly with the recipes. Try picking up different types of Keto-friendly oils to add some variety to your cooking.

Coffee and Tea

The good news is that you don't have to skip coffee if you're going on a Ketogenic Diet. The bad news is that you can't go to Starbucks anymore and order their blended coffee choices. Instead, beverages would be limited to unsweetened tea or unsweetened coffee in order to keep the sugar consumption low. Opt for organic coffee and tea products to make the most out of these powerful antioxidants.

Dark Chocolate

Yes – chocolate is still on the menu, but it is limited to just dark chocolate. Technically, this means eating chocolate that is 70 percent cacao, which would make the taste a bit bitter.

Sugar Substitutes

Later in the recipes part of this book, you might be surprised at some of the ingredients required in the list. This is because while sweeteners are an important part of food preparation, you can't just use any kind of sugar in your recipe. Remember: the typical sugar is pure carbohydrate. Even if you're not eating carbohydrates, if you're dumping lots of sugar in your food – you're not really following the Ketogenic Diet principles.

So what do you do? You find sugar substitutes. The good news is that there are LOTS of those in the market. You can get rid of the old sugar and use any of these as a good substitute.

Stevia. This is perhaps the most familiar one in this list. It's a natural sweetener derived from plants and contains very few calories. Unlike your typical sugar, stevia may actually help lower the sugar levels instead of causing it to spike. Note though that it's sweeter than actual sugar so when cooking with stevia, you'll need to lower the amount used. Typically, the ratio is 200 grams of sugar per 1 teaspoon of powdered stevia.

Sucralose. It contains zero calories and zero carbohydrates. It's actually an artificial sweetener and does not metabolize – hence the complete lack of carbohydrates. Splenda is actually a sweetener derived from sucralose. Note though that you don't want to use this as a baking substitute for sugar. Its best use is for coffee, yogurt, and oatmeal sweetening. Note though that like stevia, it's also very sweet – in fact, it's actually 600 times sweeter than the typical sugar. Use sparingly.

Erythritol. It's a naturally occurring compound that interacts with the tongue's sweet taste receptors. Hence, it mimics the taste of sugar without actually being sugar. It does contain calories, but only about 5% of the calories you'll find in the typical sugar. Note though that it doesn't dissolve very well so anything prepared with this sweetener will have a gritty feeling. This can be problematic if you're using the product for baking. As for sweetness, the typical ratio is 1 1/3 cup for 1 cup of sugar.

Xylitol. Like erythritol, xylitol is a type of sugar alcohol that's commonly used in sugar-free gum. While it still contains calories, the calories are just 3 per gram. It's a sweetener that's good for diabetic patients because it doesn't raise the sugar levels or insulin in the body. The great thing about this is that you don't have to do any computations when using it for baking, cooking, or fixing a drink. The ratio of it with sugar is 1 to 1 so you can quickly make the substitution in the recipe.

What about Condiments?

Condiments are still on the table, but they won't be as tasty as you're used to. Your options include mustard, olive oil mayonnaise, oil-based salad dressings, and unsweetened ketchup. Of all these condiments, ketchup is the one with the most sugar, so make a point of looking for one with reduced sugar content. Or maybe avoid ketchup altogether and stick to mustard?

What about Snacks?

The good news is that there are packed snacks for those who don't have the time to make it themselves. Sugarless nut butters, dried seaweeds, nuts, and sugar-free jerky are all available in stores. The nuts and seeds discussed in a previous paragraph all make for excellent snack options.

What about Labels?

Let's not fool ourselves into thinking that we can cook food every single day. The fact is that there will be days when there will be purchases for the sake of convenience. There are also instances when you'll have problems finding the right ingredients for a given recipe. Hence, you'll need to find substitutes for certain ingredients without losing the "Keto friendly" vibe of the product.

So what should be done? Well, you need to learn how to read labels. Food doesn't have to be specially made to be keto-friendly, you just have to make sure that it doesn't contain any of the unfriendly nutrients or that the carbohydrate content is low enough.

10

Buttered Cod

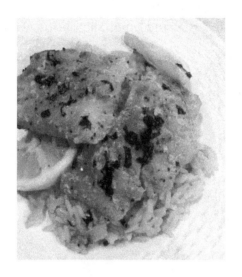

Preparation Time: 5 minutes
Cooking Time: 5 minutes
Servings: 4
Ingredients:

- 1 ½ lb. cod fillets, sliced
- 6 tablespoons butter, sliced
- ¼ teaspoon garlic powder
- ¾ teaspoon ground paprika
- Salt and pepper to taste
- Lemon slices
- Chopped parsley

Directions:

1. Mix the garlic powder, paprika, salt and pepper in a bowl.
2. Season cod pieces with seasoning mixture.
3. Add 2 tablespoons butter in a pan over medium heat.
4. Let half of the butter melt.
5. Add the cod and cook for 2 minutes per side.
6. Top with the remaining slices of butter.
7. Cook for 3 to 4 minutes.
8. Garnish with parsley and lemon slices before serving.

Nutrition:
Calories 295
Total Fat 19g
Saturated Fat 11g
Cholesterol 128mg
Sodium 236mg
Total Carbohydrate 1.5g
Dietary Fiber 0.7g
Total Sugars 0.3g
Protein 30.7g
Potassium 102mg

11

Salmon with Red Curry Sauce

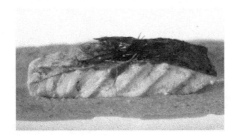

Preparation Time: 10 minutes
Cooking Time: 22 minutes
Servings: 4
Ingredients:

- 4 salmon fillets
- 2 tablespoons olive oil
- Salt and pepper to taste
- 1 ½ tablespoons red curry paste
- 1 tablespoon fresh ginger, chopped
- 14 oz. coconut cream
- 1 ½ tablespoons fish sauce

Directions:

1. Preheat your oven to 350 degrees F.
2. Cover baking sheet with foil.
3. Brush both sides of salmon fillets with olive oil and season with salt and pepper.
4. Place the salmon fillets on the baking sheet.

5. Bake salmon in the oven for 20 minutes.

6. In a pan over medium heat, mix the curry paste, ginger, coconut cream and fish sauce.

7. Sprinkle with salt and pepper.

8. Simmer for 2 minutes.

9. Pour the sauce over the salmon before serving.

Nutrition:

Calories 553

Total Fat 43.4g

Saturated Fat 24.1g

Cholesterol 78mg

Sodium 908mg

Total Carbohydrate 7.9g

Dietary Fiber 2.4g

Total Sugars 3.6g

Protein 37.3g

Potassium 982mg

12

Salmon Teriyaki

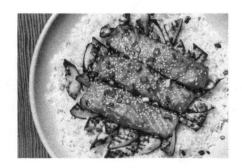

Preparation Time: 15 minutes
Cooking Time: 25 minutes
Servings: 6
Ingredients:

- 3 tablespoons sesame oil
- 2 teaspoons fish sauce
- 3 tablespoons coconut amino
- 2 teaspoons ginger, grated
- 4 cloves garlic, crushed
- 2 tablespoons xylitol
- 1 tablespoon green lime juice
- 2 teaspoons green lime zest
- Cayenne pepper to taste
- 6 salmon fillets
- 1 teaspoon arrowroot starch
- ¼ cup water
- Sesame seeds

Directions:

1. Preheat your oven to 400 degrees F.
2. Combine the sesame oil, fish sauce, coconut amino, ginger, garlic, xylitol, green lime juice, zest and cayenne pepper in a mixing bowl.
3. Create 6 packets using foil.
4. Add half of the marinade in the packets.
5. Add the salmon inside.
6. Place in the baking sheet and cook for about 20 to 25 minutes.
7. Add the remaining sauce in a pan over medium heat.
8. Dissolve arrowroot in water, and add to the sauce.
9. Simmer until the sauce has thickened.
10. Place the salmon on a serving platter and pour the sauce on top.
11. Sprinkle sesame seeds on top before serving.

Nutrition:
Calories 312
Total Fat 17.9g
Saturated Fat 2.6g
Cholesterol 78mg
Sodium 242mg
Total Carbohydrate 3.5g
Dietary Fiber 0.1g
Total Sugars 0.1g
Protein 34.8g
Potassium 706mg

13

Pesto Shrimp with Zucchini Noodles

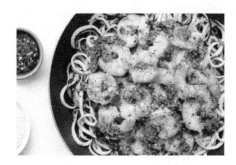

Preparation Time: 10 minutes
Cooking Time: 15 minutes
Servings: 3
Ingredients:

- Pesto sauce
- 3 cups basil leaves
- ¾ cup pine nuts
- 2 cloves garlic
- ½ lemon, juiced
- 1 teaspoon lemon zest
- Salt to taste
- ¼ cup olive oil
- Shrimp and Zoodles
- 3 zucchinis
- Salt to taste
- 1 lb. shrimp
- 2 tablespoons avocado oil

Directions:

1. Put all the pesto ingredients in a blender.
2. Blend until smooth.
3. Spiralize the zucchini into noodle form.
4. Season with salt.
5. Drain water from the zucchini noodles.
6. Season the shrimp with salt and pepper.
7. Add half of the oil in a pan over medium heat.
8. Once the oil is hot, add the shrimp and cook for 1 to 2 minutes.
9. Add the remaining oil to the pan.
10. Add the zucchini noodles and cook for 3 minutes.
11. Add the pesto and toss to coat the noodles evenly with the sauce.
12. Season with salt.

Nutrition:
Calories 304
Total Fat 22.2g
Saturated Fat 2.6g
Cholesterol 159mg
Sodium 223mg
Total Carbohydrate 8g
Dietary Fiber 2.3g
Total Sugars 2.5g
Protein 21.3g
Potassium 547mg

14

Crab Cakes

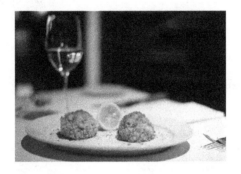

Preparation Time: 1 hour and 20 minutes
Cooking Time: 20 minutes
Servings: 8
Ingredients:

- 2 tablespoons butter
- 2 cloves garlic, minced
- ½ cup bell pepper, chopped
- 1 rib celery, chopped
- 1 shallot, chopped
- Salt and pepper to taste
- 2 tablespoons mayonnaise
- 1 egg, beaten
- 1 teaspoon mustard
- 1 tablespoon Worcestershire sauce
- 1 teaspoon hot sauce

- ½ cup Parmesan cheese, grated
- ½ cup pork rinds, crushed
- 1 lb. crabmeat
- 2 tablespoons olive oil

Directions:

- Add the butter to the pan over medium heat.
- Add the garlic, bell pepper, celery, shallot, salt and pepper.
- Cook for 10 minutes.
- In a bowl, mix the mayo, egg, Worcestershire, mustard and hot sauce.
- Add the sautéed vegetables to this mixture.
- Mix well.
- Add the cheese and pork rind.
- Fold in the crabmeat.
- Line the baking sheet with foil.
- Create patties from the mixture.
- Place the patties on the baking sheet.
- Cover the baking sheet with foil.
- Refrigerate for 1 hour.
- Fry in olive oil in a pan over medium heat.
- Cook until crispy and golden brown.

Nutrition:
Calories 150
Total Fat 9.2g
Saturated Fat 3.2g
Cholesterol 43mg
Sodium 601mg
Total Carbohydrate 10.8g
Dietary Fiber 0.5g
Total Sugars 4.6g

Protein 6.4g
Potassium 80mg

15

Tuna Salad

Preparation Time: 5 minutes
Cooking Time: 0 minute
Servings: 2
Ingredients:

- 1 cup tuna flakes
- 3 tablespoons mayonnaise
- 1 teaspoon onion flakes
- Salt and pepper to taste
- 3 cups Romaine lettuce

Directions:

1. Mix the tuna flakes, mayonnaise, onion flakes, salt and pepper in a bowl.
2. Serve with lettuce.

Nutrition:
Calories 130
Total Fat 7.8g
Saturated Fat 1.1g
Cholesterol 13mg
Sodium 206mg
Total Carbohydrate 8.5g

Dietary Fiber 0.6g
Total Sugars 2.6g
Protein 8.2g
Potassium 132mg

16

Keto Frosty

Preparation Time: 45 minutes
Cooking Time: 0 minute
Servings: 4
Ingredients:

- 1 ½ cups heavy whipping cream
- 2 tablespoons cocoa powder (unsweetened)
- 3 tablespoons Swerve
- 1 teaspoon pure vanilla extract
- Salt to taste

Directions:

1. In a bowl, combine all the ingredients.
2. Use a hand mixer and beat until you see stiff peaks forming.
3. Place the mixture in a Ziploc bag.
4. Freeze for 35 minutes.
5. Serve in bowls or dishes.

Nutrition:
Calories 164
Total Fat 17g
Saturated Fat 10.6g
Cholesterol 62mg

Sodium 56mg
Total Carbohydrate 2.9g
Dietary Fiber 0.8g
Total Sugars 0.2g
Protein 1.4g
Potassium 103mg

17

Keto Shake

Preparation Time: 15 minutes
Cooking Time: 0 minute
Serving: 1
Ingredients:

- ¾ cup almond milk
- ½ cup ice
- 2 tablespoons almond butter
- 2 tablespoons cocoa powder (unsweetened)
- 2 tablespoons Swerve
- 1 tablespoon chia seeds
- 2 tablespoons hemp seeds
- ½ tablespoon vanilla extract
- Salt to taste

Directions:

1. Blend all the ingredients in a food processor.
2. Chill in the refrigerator before serving.

Nutrition:
Calories 104
Total Fat 9.5g
Saturated Fat 5.1g

Cholesterol 0mg
Sodium 24mg
Total Carbohydrate 3.6g
Dietary Fiber 1.4g
Total Sugars 1.1g
Protein 2.9g
Potassium 159mg

18

Keto Fat Bombs

Preparation Time: 30 minutes
Cooking Time: 0 minute
Servings: 10
Ingredients:

- 8 tablespoons butter
- ¼ cup Swerve
- ½ teaspoon vanilla extract
- Salt to taste
- 2 cups almond flour
- 2/3 cup chocolate chips

Directions:

1. In a bowl, beat the butter until fluffy.
2. Stir in the sugar, salt and vanilla.
3. Mix well.
4. Add the almond flour.
5. Fold in the chocolate chips.
6. Cover the bowl with cling wrap and refrigerate for 20 minutes.
7. Create balls from the dough.

Nutrition:
Calories 176

Total Fat 15.2g
Saturated Fat 8.4g
Cholesterol 27mg
Sodium 92mg
Total Carbohydrate 12.9g
Dietary Fiber 1g
Total Sugars 10.8g
Protein 2.2g
Potassium 45mg

19

Avocado Ice Pops

Preparation Time: 20 minutes
Cooking Time: 0 minute
Servings: 10
Ingredients:

- 3 avocados
- ¼ cup lime juice
- 3 tablespoons Swerve
- ¾ cup coconut milk
- 1 tablespoon coconut oil
- 1 cup keto friendly chocolate

Directions:

1. Add all the ingredients except the oil and chocolate in a blender.
2. Blend until smooth.
3. Pour the mixture into the popsicle mold.
4. Freeze overnight.
5. In a bowl, mix oil and chocolate chips.
6. Melt in the microwave. And then let cool.
7. Dunk the avocado popsicles into the chocolate before serving.

Nutrition:
Calories 176

Total Fat 17.4g
Saturated Fat 7.5g
Cholesterol 0mg
Sodium 6mg
Total Carbohydrate 10.8g
Dietary Fiber 4.5g
Total Sugars 5.4g
Protein 1.6g
Potassium 341mg

20

Carrot Balls

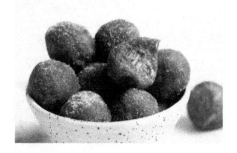

Preparation Time: 1 hour and 10 minutes
Cooking Time: 0 minute
Servings: 8
Ingredients:

- 8 oz. block cream cheese
- ¾ cup coconut flour
- ½ teaspoon pure vanilla extract
- 1 teaspoon stevia
- ¼ teaspoon ground nutmeg
- 1 teaspoon cinnamon
- 1 cup carrots, grated
- 1/2 cup pecans, chopped
- 1 cup coconut, shredded

Directions:

Use a hand mixer to beat the cream cheese, coconut flour, vanilla, stevia, nutmeg and cinnamon.

Fold in the carrots and pecans.

Form into balls.

Refrigerate for 1 hour.

Roll into shredded coconut before serving.

Nutrition:

Calories 390

Total Fat 35g

Saturated Fat 17g

Cholesterol 60mg

Sodium 202mg

Total Carbohydrate 17.2g

Dietary Fiber 7.8g

Total Sugars 6g

Protein 7.8g

Potassium 154mg

21

Coconut Crack Bars

Preparation Time: 2 minutes
Cooking Time: 3 minutes
Servings: 20
Ingredients:

- 3 cups coconut flakes (unsweetened)
- 1 cup coconut oil
- ¼ cup maple syrup

Directions:

1. Line a baking sheet with parchment paper.
2. Put coconut in a bowl.
3. Add the oil and syrup.
4. Mix well.
5. Pour the mixture into the pan.
6. Refrigerate until firm.
7. Slice into bars before serving.

Nutrition:
Calories 147
Total Fat 14.9g
Saturated Fat 13g
Cholesterol 0mg

Sodium 3mg
Total Carbohydrate 4.5g
Dietary Fiber 1.1g
Total Sugars 3.1g
Protein 0.4g
Potassium 51mg

22

Strawberry Ice Cream

Preparation Time: 1 hour and 20 minutes
Cooking Time: 0 minute
Servings: 4
Ingredients:

- 17 oz. coconut milk
- 16 oz. frozen strawberries
- ¾ cup Swerve
- ½ cup fresh strawberries

Directions:

1. Put all the ingredients except fresh strawberries in a blender.
2. Pulse until smooth.
3. Put the mixture in an ice cream maker.
4. Use ice cream maker according to directions.
5. Add the fresh strawberries a few minutes before the ice cream is done.
6. Freeze for 1 hour before serving.

Nutrition:
Calories 320
Total Fat 28.8g
Saturated Fat 25.5g

Cholesterol 0mg
Sodium 18mg
Total Carbohydrate 25.3g
Dietary Fiber 5.3g
Total Sugars 19.1g
Protein 2.9g
Potassium 344mg

23

Key Lime Pudding

Preparation Time: 20 minutes
Cooking Time: 1 hour and 15 minutes
Servings: 2
Ingredients:

- 1 cup hot water
- 2/4 cup erythrytol syrup
- 6 drops stevia
- 1 teaspoon almond extract
- 1 teaspoon vanilla extract
- ¼ teaspoon Xanthan gum powder
- 2 ripe avocados, sliced
- 1 ½ oz. lime juice
- 3 tablespoons coconut oil
- Salt to taste

Directions:

1. Add water, erythritol, stevia, almond extract and vanilla extract to a pot.
2. Bring to a boil.
3. Simmer until the syrup has been reduced and has thickened.
4. Turn the heat off.
5. Add the gum powder.

6. Mix until thickened.
7. Add the avocado into a food processor.
8. Add the rest of the ingredients.
9. Pulse until smooth.
10. Place the mixture in ramekins.
11. Refrigerate for 1 hour.
12. Pour the syrup over the pudding before serving.

Nutrition:
Calories 299
Total Fat 29.8g
Saturated Fat 12.9g
Cholesterol 0mg
Sodium 47mg
Total Carbohydrate 9.7g
Dietary Fiber 6.8g
Total Sugars 0.8g
Protein 2g
Potassium 502mg

24

Chicken, Bacon and Avocado Cloud Sandwiches

Preparation Time: 10 minutes
Cooking Time: 25 minutes
Servings: 6
Ingredients:

- For cloud bread
- 3 large eggs
- 4 oz. cream cheese
- ½ tablespoon. ground psyllium husk powder
- ½ teaspoon baking powder
- A pinch of salt
- To assemble sandwich
- 6 slices of bacon, cooked and chopped
- 6 slices pepper Jack cheese
- ½ avocado, sliced
- 1 cup cooked chicken breasts, shredded
- 3 tablespoons. mayonnaise

Directions:

1. Preheat your oven to 300 degrees.
2. Prepare a baking sheet by lining it with parchment paper.

3. Separate the egg whites and egg yolks, and place into separate bowls.
4. Whisk the egg whites until very stiff. Set aside.
5. Combined egg yolks and cream cheese.
6. Add the psyllium husk powder and baking powder to the egg yolk mixture. Gently fold in.
7. Add the egg whites into the egg mixture and gently fold in.
8. Dollop the mixture onto the prepared baking sheet to create 12 cloud bread. Use a spatula to gently spread the circles around to form ½-inch thick pieces.
9. Bake for 25 minutes or until the tops are golden brown.
10. Allow the cloud bread to cool completely before serving. Can be refrigerated for up to 3 days of frozen for up to 3 months. If food prepping, place a layer of parchment paper between each bread slice to avoid having them getting stuck together. Simply toast in the oven for 5 minutes when it is time to serve.
11. To assemble sandwiches, place mayonnaise on one side of one cloud bread. Layer with the remaining sandwich ingredients and top with another slice of cloud bread.

Nutrition:
Calories: 333 kcal
Carbs: 5g
Fat: 26g
Protein: 19.9g

25

Roasted Lemon Chicken Sandwich

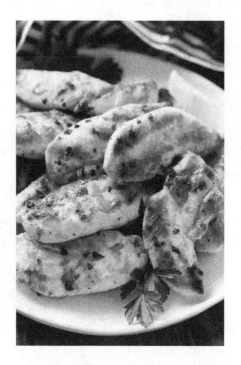

Preparation Time: 15 minutes
Cooking Time: 1 hour 30 minutes
Servings: 12
Ingredients:

- 1 kg whole chicken
- 5 tablespoons. butter

- 1 lemon, cut into wedges
- 1 tablespoon. garlic powder
- Salt and pepper to taste
- 2 tablespoons. mayonnaise
- Keto-friendly bread

Directions:

1. Preheat the oven to 350 degrees F.
2. Grease a deep baking dish with butter.
3. Ensure that the chicken is patted dry and that the gizzards have been removed.
4. Combine the butter, garlic powder, salt and pepper.
5. Rub the entire chicken with it, including in the cavity.
6. Place the lemon and onion inside the chicken and place the chicken in the prepared baking dish.
7. Bake for about 1½ hours, depending on the size of the chicken.
8. Baste the chicken often with the drippings. If the drippings begin to dry, add water. The chicken is done when a thermometer, insert it into the thickest part of the thigh reads 165 degrees F or when the clear juices run when the thickest part of the thigh is pierced.
9. Allow the chicken to cool before slicing.
10. To assemble sandwich, shred some of the breast meat and mix with the mayonnaise. Place the mixture between the two bread slices.
11. To save the chicken, refrigerated for up to 5 days or freeze for up to 1 month.

Nutrition:
Calories: 214 kcal
Carbs: 1.6 g
Fat: 11.8 g

Protein: 24.4 g.

26

Keto-Friendly Skillet Pepperoni Pizza

Preparation Time: 10 minutes
Cooking Time: 6 minutes
Servings: 4
Ingredients:
For Crust
½ cup almond flour
½ teaspoon baking powder
8 large egg whites, whisked into stiff peaks
Salt and pepper to taste
Toppings
3 tablespoons. Unsweetened tomato sauce
½ cup shredded cheddar cheese
½ cup pepperoni
Directions
Gently incorporate the almond flour into the egg whites. Ensure that no lumps remain.

Stir in the remaining crust ingredients.

Heat a nonstick skillet over medium heat. Spray with nonstick spray.

Pour the batter into the heated skillet to cover the bottom of the skillet.

Cover the skillet with a lid and cook the pizza crust to cook for about 4 minutes or until bubbles that appear on the top.

Flip the dough and add the toppings, starting with the tomato sauce and ending with the pepperoni

Cook the pizza for 2 more minutes.

Allow the pizza to cool slightly before serving.

Can be stored in the refrigerator for up to 5 days and frozen for up to 1 month.

Nutrition:

Calories: 175 kcal

Carbs: 1.9 g

Fat: 12 g

Protein: 14.3 g.

27

Cheesy Chicken Cauliflower

Preparation Time: 5 minutes
Cooking Time: 10 minutes
Servings: 4
Ingredients:

- 2 cups cauliflower florets, chopped
- ½ cup red bell pepper, chopped
- 1 cup roasted chicken, shredded (Lunch Recipes: Roasted Lemon Chicken Sandwich)
- ¼ cup shredded cheddar cheese
- 1 tablespoon. butter
- 1 tablespoon. sour cream
- Salt and pepper to taste

Directions:

1. Stir fry the cauliflower and peppers in the butter over medium heat until the veggies are tender.
2. Add the chicken and cook until the chicken is warmed through.
3. Add the remaining ingredients and stir until the cheese is melted.
4. Serve warm.

Nutrition:
Calories: 144 kcal

Carbs: 4 g
Fat: 8.5 g
Protein: 13.2 g.

28

Chicken Soup

Preparation Time: 10 minutes
Cooking Time: 25 minutes
Servings: 6
Ingredients:

- 4 cups roasted chicken, shredded (Lunch Recipes: Roasted Lemon Chicken Sandwich)
- 2 tablespoons. butter
- 2 celery stalks, chopped
- 1 cup mushrooms, sliced
- 4 cups green cabbage, sliced into strips
- 2 garlic cloves, minced
- 6 cups chicken broth
- 1 carrot, sliced
- Salt and pepper to taste
- 1 tablespoon. garlic powder
- 1 tablespoon. onion powder

Directions:

1. Sauté the celery, mushrooms and garlic in the butter in a pot over medium heat for 4 minutes.
2. Add broth, carrots, garlic powder, onion powder, salt, and pepper.

3. Simmer for 10 minutes or until the vegetables are tender.
4. Add the chicken and cabbage and simmer for another 10 minutes or until the cabbage is tender.
5. Serve warm.
6. Can be refrigerated for up to 3 days or frozen for up to 1 month.

Nutrition:
Calories: 279 kcal
Carbs: 7.5 g
Fat: 12.3 g
Protein: 33.4 g.

29

Chicken Avocado Salad

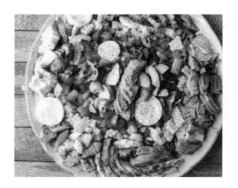

Preparation Time: 7 minutes
Cooking Time: 10 minutes
Servings: 4
Ingredients:

- 1 cup roasted chicken, shredded (Lunch Recipes: Roasted Lemon Chicken Sandwich)
- 1 bacon strip, cooked and chopped
- 1/2 medium avocado, chopped
- ¼ cup cheddar cheese, grated
- 1 hard-boiled egg, chopped
- 1 cup romaine lettuce, chopped
- 1 tablespoon. olive oil
- 1 tablespoon. apple cider vinegar
- Salt and pepper to taste

Directions:

1. Create the dressing by mixing apple cider vinegar, oil, salt and pepper.
2. Combine all the other ingredients in a mixing bowl.
3. Drizzle with the dressing and toss.
4. Can be refrigerated for up to 3 days.

Nutrition:
Calories: 220 kcal
Carbs: 2.8 g
Fat: 16.7 g
Protein: 14.8 g.

30

Chicken Broccoli Dinner

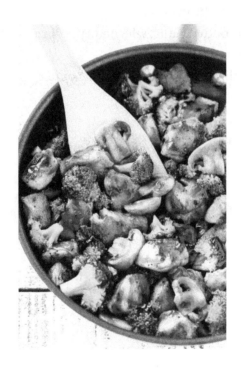

Preparation Time: 10 minutes
Cooking Time: 5 minutes
Servings: 1
Ingredients:

- 1 roasted chicken leg (Lunch Recipes: Roasted Lemon Chicken Sandwich)
- ½ cup broccoli florets

- ½ tablespoon. unsalted butter, softened
- 2 garlic cloves, minced
- Salt and pepper to taste

Directions:

1. Boil the broccoli in lightly salted water for 5 minutes. Drain the water from the pot and keep the broccoli in the pot. Keep the lid on to keep the broccoli warm.
2. Mix all the butter, garlic, salt and pepper in a small bowl to create garlic butter.
3. Place the chicken, broccoli and garlic butter.

Nutrition:
Calories: 257 kcal
Carbs: 5.1 g
Fat: 14 g
Protein: 27.4 g.

31

Easy Meatballs

Preparation Time: 10 minutes
Cooking Time: 20 minutes
Servings: 4
Ingredients:

- 1 lb. ground beef
- 1 egg, beaten
- Salt and pepper to taste
- 1 teaspoon garlic powder
- 1 teaspoon onion powder
- 2 tablespoons. butter
- ¼ cup mayonnaise
- ¼ cup pickled jalapeños
- 1 cup cheddar cheese, grated

Directions

1. Combine the cheese, mayonnaise, pickled jalapenos, salt, pepper, garlic powder and onion powder in a large mixing bowl.
2. Add the beef and egg and combine using clean hands.
3. Form large meatballs. Makes about 12.
4. Fry the meatballs in the butter over medium heat for about 4 minutes on each side or until golden brown.
5. Serve warm with a keto-friendly side.

6. The meatball mixture can also be used to make a meatloaf. Just preheat your oven to 400 degrees F, press the mixture into a loaf pan and bake for about 30 minutes or until the top is golden brown.

7. Can be refrigerated for up to 5 days or frozen for up to 3 months.

Nutrition:
Calories: 454 kcal
Carbs: 5 g
Fat: 28.2 g
Protein: 43.2 g.

32

Chicken Casserole

Preparation Time: 10 minutes
Cooking Time: 40 minutes
Servings: 8
Ingredients:

- 1 lb. boneless chicken breasts, cut into 1" cubes
- 2 tablespoons. butter
- 4 tablespoons. green pesto
- 1 cup heavy whipping cream
- ¼ cup green bell peppers, diced
- 1 cup feta cheese, diced
- 1 garlic clove, minced
- Salt and pepper to taste

Directions

1. Preheat your oven to 400 degrees F.
2. Season the chicken with salt and pepper then batch fry in the butter until golden brown.
3. Place the fried chicken pieces in a baking dish. Add the feta cheese, garlic and bell peppers.
4. Combine the pesto and heavy cream in a bowl. Pour on top of the chicken mixture and spread with a spatula.

5. Bake for 30 minutes or until the casserole is light brown around the edges.

6. Serve warm.

7. Can be refrigerated for up to 5 days and frozen for 2 weeks.

Nutrition:
Calories: 294 kcal
Carbs: 1.7 g
Fat: 22.7 g
Protein: 20.1 g.

33

Lemon Baked Salmon

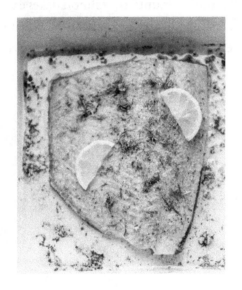

Preparation Time: 10 minutes
Cooking Time: 30 minutes
Servings: 4
Ingredients:

- 1 lb. salmon
- 1 tablespoon. olive oil
- Salt and pepper to taste
- 1 tablespoon. butter
- 1 lemon, thinly sliced
- 1 tablespoon. lemon juice

Directions:

1. Preheat your oven to 400 degrees F.
2. Grease a baking dish with the olive oil and place the salmon skin-side down.
3. Season the salmon with salt and pepper then top with the lemon slices.
4. Slice half the butter and place over the salmon.
5. Bake for 20minutes or until the salmon flakes easily.
6. Melt the remaining butter in a saucepan. When it starts to bubble, remove from heat and allow to cool before adding the lemon juice.
7. Drizzle the lemon butter over the salmon and Serve warm.

Nutrition:
Calories: 211 kcal
Carbs: 1.5 g
Fat: 13.5 g
Protein: 22.2 g.

34

Italian Sausage Stacks

Preparation Time: 10 minutes
Cooking Time: 25 minutes
Servings: 3
Ingredients:

- 6 Italian sausage patties
- 4 tablespoon olive oil
- 2 ripe avocados, pitted
- 2 teaspoon fresh lime juice
- Salt and black pepper to taste
- 6 fresh eggs
- Red pepper flakes to garnish

Directions:

1. In a skillet, warm the oil over medium heat and fry the sausage patties about 8 minutes until lightly browned and firm. Remove the patties to a plate.
2. Spoon the avocado into a bowl, mash with the lime juice, and season with salt and black pepper. Spread the mash on the sausages.
3. Boil 3 cups of water in a wide pan over high heat, and reduce to simmer (don't boil).
4. Crack each egg into a small bowl and gently put the egg into the simmering water; poach for 2 to 3 minutes. Use a perforated

spoon to remove from the water on a paper towel to dry. Repeat with the other 5 eggs. Top each stack with a poached egg, sprinkle with chili flakes, salt, black pepper, and chives. Serve with turnip wedges.

Nutrition:
Kcal 378,
Fat 23g,
Net Carbs 5g,
Protein 16g

35

Baked Salmon

Preparation Time: 10 minutes
Cooking Time: 10 minutes
Servings: 4
Ingredients:

- Cooking spray
- 3 cloves garlic, minced
- ¼ cup butter
- 1 teaspoon lemon zest
- 2 tablespoons lemon juice
- 4 salmon fillets
- Salt and pepper to taste
- 2 tablespoons parsley, chopped

Directions:

1. Preheat your oven to 425 degrees F.
2. Grease the pan with cooking spray.
3. In a bowl, mix the garlic, butter, and lemon zest and lemon juice.
4. Sprinkle salt and pepper on salmon fillets.
5. Drizzle with the lemon butter sauce.
6. Bake in the oven for 12 minutes.
7. Garnish with parsley before serving.

Nutrition:
Calories 345
Total Fat 22.7g
Saturated Fat 8.9g
Cholesterol 109mg
Sodium 163mg
Total Carbohydrate 1.2g
Dietary Fiber 0.2g
Total Sugars 0.2g
Protein 34.9g
Potassium 718mg

36

Tuna Patties

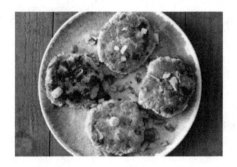

Preparation Time: 10 minutes
Cooking Time: 10 minutes
Servings: 8
Ingredients:

- 20 oz. canned tuna flakes
- ¼ cup almond flour
- 1 egg, beaten
- 2 tablespoons fresh dill, chopped
- 2 stalks green onion, chopped
- Salt and pepper to taste
- 1 tablespoon lemon zest
- ¼ cup mayonnaise
- 1 tablespoon lemon juice
- 2 tablespoons avocado oil

Directions:

1. Combine all the ingredients except avocado oil, lemon juice and avocado oil in a large bowl.
2. Form 8 patties from the mixture.
3. In a pan over medium heat, add the oil.
4. Once the oil starts to sizzle, cook the tuna patties for 3 to 4 minutes per side.
5. Drain each patty on a paper towel.
6. Spread mayo on top and drizzle with lemon juice before serving.

Nutrition:
Calories 101
Total Fat 4.9g
Saturated Fat 1.2g
Cholesterol 47mg
Sodium 243mg
Total Carbohydrate 3.1g
Dietary Fiber 0.5g
Total Sugars 0.7g
Protein 12.3g
Potassium 60mg

37

Cauliflower Mash

Preparation Time: 10 minutes
Cooking Time: 5 minutes
Servings: 8
Ingredients:

- 4 cups cauliflower florets, chopped
- 1 cup grated parmesan cheese
- 6 tablespoons. butter
- ½ lemon, juice and zest
- Salt and pepper to taste

Directions:

1. Boil the cauliflower in lightly salted water over high heat for 5 minutes or until the florets are tender but still firm.
2. Strain the cauliflower in a colander and add the cauliflower to a food processor
3. Add the remaining ingredients and pulse the mixture to a smooth and creamy consistency
4. Serve with protein like salmon, chicken or meatballs.
5. Can be refrigerated for up to 3 days.

Nutrition:
Calories: 101 kcal

Carbs: 3.1 g
Fat: 9.5 g
Protein: 2.2 g.

38

Almond Waffles with Cinnamon Cream

Preparation Time: 10 minutes
Cooking Time: 25 minutes
Servings: 3
Ingredients:

- For the Spread
- 8 oz. cream cheese, at room temperature
- 1 teaspoon cinnamon powder
- 3 tablespoon swerve brown sugar
- Cinnamon powder for garnishing
- For the Waffles
- 5 tablespoon melted butter
- 1 ½ cups unsweetened almond milk
- 7 large eggs
- ¼ teaspoon liquid stevia
- ½ teaspoon baking powder
- 1 ½ cups almond flour

Directions:

1. Combine the cream cheese, cinnamon, and swerve with a hand mixer until smooth. Cover and chill until ready to use.

2. To make the waffles, whisk the butter, milk, and eggs in a medium bowl. Add the stevia and baking powder and mix. Stir in the almond flour and combine until no lumps exist. Let the batter sit for 5 minutes to thicken. Spritz a waffle iron with a non-stick cooking spray.

3. Ladle a ¼ cup of the batter into the waffle iron and cook according to the manufacturer's instructions until golden, about 10 minutes in total. Repeat with the remaining batter.

4. Slice the waffles into quarters; apply the cinnamon spread in between each of two waffles and snap. Sprinkle with cinnamon powder and serve.

Nutrition:
Kcal 307,
Fat 24g,
Net Carbs 8g,
Protein 12g

39

Grilled Mahi with Lemon Butter Sauce

Preparation Time: 20 minutes
Cooking Time: 10 minutes
Servings: 6
Ingredients:

- 6 mahi fillets
- Salt and pepper to taste
- 2 tablespoons olive oil
- 6 tablespoons butter
- ¼ onion, minced
- ½ teaspoon garlic, minced
- ¼ cup chicken stock
- 1 tablespoon lemon juice

Directions:

1. Preheat your grill to medium heat.
2. Season fish fillets with salt and pepper.
3. Coat both sides with olive oil.
4. Grill for 3 to 4 minutes per side.
5. Place fish on a serving platter.
6. In a pan over medium heat, add the butter and let it melt.
7. Add the onion and sauté for 2 minutes.

8. Add the garlic and cook for 30 seconds.
9. Pour in the chicken stock.
10. Simmer until the stock has been reduced to half.
11. Add the lemon juice.
12. Pour the sauce over the grilled fish fillets.

Nutrition:
Calories 234
Total Fat 17.2g
Saturated Fat 8.3g
Cholesterol 117mg
Sodium 242mg
Total Carbohydrate 0.6g
Dietary Fiber 0.1g
Total Sugars 0.3g
Protein 19.1g
Potassium 385mg

40

Shrimp Scampi

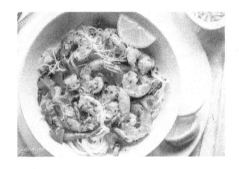

Preparation Time: 15 minutes
Cooking Time: 10 minutes
Servings: 6
Ingredients:

- 2 tablespoons olive oil
- 2 tablespoons butter
- 1 tablespoon garlic, minced
- ½ cup dry white wine
- ¼ teaspoon red pepper flakes
- Salt and pepper to taste
- 2 lb. large shrimp, peeled and deveined
- ¼ cup fresh parsley, chopped
- 1 teaspoon lemon zest
- 2 tablespoons lemon juice
- 3 cups spaghetti squash, cooked

Directions:

1. In a pan over medium heat, add the oil and butter.
2. Cook the garlic for 2 minutes.
3. Pour in the wine.
4. Add the red pepper flakes, salt and pepper.
5. Cook for 2 minutes.
6. Add the shrimp.
7. Cook for 2 to 3 minutes.
8. Remove from the stove.
9. Add the parsley, lemon zest and lemon juice.
10. Serve on top of spaghetti squash.

Nutrition:
Calories 232
Total Fat 8.9g
Saturated Fat 3.2g
Cholesterol 226mg
Sodium 229mg
Total Carbohydrate 7.6g
Dietary Fiber 0.2g
Total Sugars 0.3g
Protein 28.9g
Potassium 104mg

Dark Chocolate Smoothie

Preparation Time: 10 minutes
Cooking Time: 25 minutes
Servings: 3
Ingredients:

- 8 pecans
- ¾ cup coconut milk
- ¼ cup water
- 1 ½ cups watercress
- 2 teaspoon vegan protein powder
- 1 tablespoon chia seeds
- 1 tablespoon unsweetened cocoa powder
- 4 fresh dates, pitted

Directions

1. In a blender, add all ingredients and process until creamy and uniform. Place into two glasses and chill before serving.

Nutrition:
Kcal 335;
Fat: 31.7g
Net Carbs: 12.7g,
Protein: 7g

Five Greens Smoothie

Preparation Time: 10 minutes
Cooking Time: 25 minutes
Servings: 3
Ingredients:

- 6 kale leaves, chopped
- 3 stalks celery, chopped
- 1 ripe avocado, skinned, pitted, sliced
- 1 cup ice cubes
- 2 cups spinach, chopped
- 1 large cucumber, peeled and chopped
- Chia seeds to garnish

Directions:

1. In a blender, add the kale, celery, avocado, and ice cubes, and blend for 45 seconds. Add the spinach and cucumber, and process for another 45 seconds until smooth.
2. Pour the smoothie into glasses, garnish with chia seeds and serve the drink immediately.

Nutrition:
Kcal 124,
Fat 7.8g,

Net Carbs 2.9g,
Protein 3.2g

43

Smoked Salmon Rolls with Dill Cream Cheese

Preparation Time: 10 minutes
Cooking Time: 25 minutes
Servings: 3
Ingredients:

- 3 tablespoon cream cheese, softened
- 1 small lemon, zested and juiced
- 3 teaspoon chopped fresh dill
- Salt and black pepper to taste
- 3 (7-inch) low carb tortillas
- 6 slices smoked salmon

Directions

1. In a bowl, mix the cream cheese, lemon juice, zest, dill, salt, and black pepper.
2. Lay each tortilla on a plastic wrap (just wide enough to cover the tortilla), spread with cream cheese mixture, and top each (one) with two salmon slices. Roll up the tortillas and secure both ends by twisting.
3. Refrigerate for 2 hours, remove plastic, cut off both ends of each wrap, and cut wraps into wheels.

Nutrition:
Kcal 250,
Fat 16g,
Net Carbs 7g,
Protein 18g

44

Pan-Seared Halibut with Citrus Butter Sauce

Preparation Time: 10 minutes
Cooking Time: 15 minutes
Servings: 3
Ingredients:

- 4 (5-ounce) halibut fillets, each about 1 inch thick
- Sea salt
- Freshly ground black pepper
- ¼ cup butter
- 2 teaspoons minced garlic
- 1 shallot, minced
- 3 tablespoons dry white wine
- 1 tablespoon freshly squeezed lemon juice
- 1 tablespoon freshly squeezed orange juice
- 2 teaspoons chopped fresh parsley
- 2 tablespoons olive oil

Directions:

1. Pat the fish dry with paper towels and then lightly season the fillets with salt and pepper. Set aside on a paper towel–lined plate.
2. Place a small saucepan over medium heat and melt the butter.
3. Sauté the garlic and shallot until tender, about 3 minutes.

4. Whisk in the white wine, lemon juice, and orange juice and bring the sauce to a simmer, cooking until it thickens slightly, about 2 minutes.

5. Remove the sauce from the heat and stir in the parsley; set aside.

6. Place a large skillet over medium-high heat and add the olive oil.

7. Panfry the fish until lightly browned and just cooked through, turning them over once, about 10 minutes in total.

8. Serve the fish immediately with a spoonful of sauce for each.

Nutrition:
Calories: 319
Fat: 26g
Protein: 22g
Carbohydrates: 2g
Fiber: 0g

45

Lemon Butter Chicken

Preparation Time: 10 minutes
Cooking Time: 40 minutes
Servings: 4
Ingredients:

- 4 bone-in, skin-on chicken thighs
- Sea salt
- Freshly ground black pepper
- 2 tablespoons butter, divided
- 2 teaspoons minced garlic
- ½ cup Herbed Chicken Stock
- ½ cup heavy (whipping) cream
- Juice of ½ lemon

Directions:

1. Preheat the oven to 400°F.
2. Lightly season the chicken thighs with salt and pepper.
3. Place a large ovenproof skillet over medium-high heat and add 1 tablespoon of butter.
4. Brown the chicken thighs until golden on both sides, about 6 minutes in total. Remove the thighs to a plate and set aside.
5. Add the remaining 1 tablespoon of butter and sauté the garlic until translucent, about 2 minutes.

6. Whisk in the chicken stock, heavy cream, and lemon juice.
7. Bring the sauce to a boil and then return the chicken to the skillet.
8. Place the skillet in the oven, covered, and braise until the chicken is cooked through, about 30 minutes.

Nutrition:
Calories: 294
Fat: 26g
Protein: 12g
Carbohydrates: 4g
Fiber: 1g

46

Simple Fish Curry

Preparation Time: 10 minutes
Cooking Time: 25 minutes
Servings: 4
Ingredients:

- 2 tablespoons coconut oil
- 1½ tablespoons grated fresh ginger
- 2 teaspoons minced garlic
- 1 tablespoon curry powder
- ½ teaspoon ground cumin
- 2 cups coconut milk
- 16 ounces firm white fish, cut into 1-inch chunks
- 1 cup shredded kale
- 2 tablespoons chopped cilantro

Directions:

1. Place a large saucepan over medium heat and melt the coconut oil.
2. Sauté the ginger and garlic until lightly browned, about 2 minutes.
3. Stir in the curry powder and cumin and sauté until very fragrant, about 2 minutes.
4. Stir in the coconut milk and bring the liquid to a boil.

5. Reduce the heat to low and simmer for about 5 minutes to infuse the milk with the spices.
6. Add the fish and cook until the fish is cooked through, about 10 minutes.
7. Stir in the kale and cilantro and simmer until wilted, about 2 minutes.
8. Serve.

Nutrition:
Calories: 416
Fat: 31g
Protein: 26g
Carbohydrates: 5g
Fiber: 1g]

47

Roasted Salmon with Avocado Salsa

Preparation Time: 15 minutes
Cooking Time: 12 minutes
Servings: 4
Ingredients:

- For the Salsa
- 1 avocado, peeled, pitted, and diced
- 1 scallion, white and green parts, chopped
- ½ cup halved cherry tomatoes
- Juice of 1 lemon
- Zest of 1 lemon
- For the Fish
- 1 teaspoon ground cumin
- ½ teaspoon ground coriander
- ½ teaspoon onion powder
- ¼ teaspoon sea salt
- Pinch freshly ground black pepper
- Pinch cayenne pepper
- 4 (4-ounce) boneless, skinless salmon fillets
- 2 tablespoons olive oil

Directions:

1. To Make the Salsa
2. In a small bowl, stir together the avocado, scallion, tomatoes, lemon juice, and lemon zest until mixed.
3. Set aside.
4. To Make the Fish
5. Preheat the oven to 400°F. Line a baking sheet with aluminum foil and set aside.
6. In a small bowl, stir together the cumin, coriander, onion powder, salt, black pepper, and cayenne until well mixed.
7. Rub the salmon fillets with the spice mix and place them on the baking sheet.
8. Drizzle the fillets with the olive oil and roast the fish until it is just cooked through, about 15 minutes.
9. Serve the salmon topped with the avocado salsa.

Nutrition:
Calories: 320
Fat: 26g
Protein: 22g
Carbohydrates: 4g
Fiber: 3g

48

Sole Asiago

Preparation Time: 10 minutes
Cooking Time: 8 minutes
Servings: 4
Ingredients:

- 4 (4-ounce) sole fillets
- ¾ cup ground almonds
- ¼ cup Asiago cheese
- 2 eggs, beaten
- 2½ tablespoons melted coconut oil

Directions:

1. Preheat the oven to 350°F. Line a baking sheet with parchment paper and set aside.
2. Pat the fish dry with paper towels.
3. Stir together the ground almonds and cheese in a small bowl.
4. Place the bowl with the beaten eggs in it next to the almond mixture.
5. Dredge a sole fillet in the beaten egg and then press the fish into the almond mixture so it is completely coated. Place on the baking sheet and repeat until all the fillets are breaded.
6. Brush both sides of each piece of fish with the coconut oil.
7. Bake the sole until it is cooked through, about 8 minutes in total.

8. Serve immediately.

Nutrition:
Calories: 406
Fat: 31g
Protein: 29g
Carbohydrates: 6g
Fiber: 3g

49

Baked Coconut Haddock

Preparation Time: 10 minutes
Cooking Time: 12 minutes
Servings: 4
Ingredients:

- 4 (5-ounce) boneless haddock fillets
- Sea salt
- Freshly ground black pepper
- 1 cup shredded unsweetened coconut
- ¼ cup ground hazelnuts
- 2 tablespoons coconut oil, melted

Directions:

1. Preheat the oven to 400°F. Line a baking sheet with parchment paper and set aside.
2. Pat the fillets very dry with paper towels and lightly season them with salt and pepper.
3. Stir together the shredded coconut and hazelnuts in a small bowl.
4. Dredge the fish fillets in the coconut mixture so that both sides of each piece are thickly coated.
5. Place the fish on the baking sheet and lightly brush both sides of each piece with the coconut oil.

6. Bake the haddock until the topping is golden and the fish flakes easily with a fork, about 12 minutes total.

7. Serve.

8. PREP TIP the breading of the fish can be done ahead, up to 1 day, if you just want to pop the fish in the oven when you get home. Place the breaded fish on the baking sheet and cover it with plastic wrap in the refrigerator until you wish to bake it.

Nutrition:

Calories: 299

Fat: 24g

Protein: 20g

Carbohydrates: 4g

Fiber: 3g

50

Cheesy Garlic Salmon

Preparation Time: 15 minutes
Cooking Time: 12 minutes
Servings: 4
Ingredients:

- ½ cup Asiago cheese
- 2 tablespoons freshly squeezed lemon juice
- 2 tablespoons butter, at room temperature
- 2 teaspoons minced garlic
- 1 teaspoon chopped fresh basil
- 1 teaspoon chopped fresh oregano
- 4 (5-ounce) salmon fillets
- 1 tablespoon olive oil

Directions:

1. Preheat the oven to 350°F. Line a baking sheet with parchment paper and set aside.
2. In a small bowl, stir together the Asiago cheese, lemon juice, butter, garlic, basil, and oregano.
3. Pat the salmon dry with paper towels and place the fillets on the baking sheet skin-side down. Divide the topping evenly between the fillets and spread it across the fish using a knife or the back of a spoon.

4. Drizzle the fish with the olive oil and bake until the topping is golden and the fish is just cooked through, about 12 minutes.
5. Serve.

Nutrition:
Calories: 357
Fat: 28g
Protein: 24g
Carbohydrates: 2g
Fiber: 0g

51

Chicken Bacon Burgers

Preparation Time: 10 minutes
Cooking Time: 25 minutes
Servings: 4
Ingredients:

- 1-pound ground chicken
- 8 bacon slices, chopped
- ¼ cup ground almonds
- 1 teaspoon chopped fresh basil
- ¼ teaspoon sea salt
- Pinch freshly ground black pepper
- 2 tablespoons coconut oil
- 4 large lettuce leaves
- 1 avocado, peeled, pitted, and sliced

Directions:

1. Preheat the oven to 350°F. Line a baking sheet with parchment paper and set aside.
2. In a medium bowl, combine the chicken, bacon, ground almonds, basil, salt, and pepper until well mixed.
3. Form the mixture into 6 equal patties.
4. Place a large skillet over medium-high heat and add the coconut oil.

5. Pan sear the chicken patties until brown on both sides, about 6 minutes in total.

6. Place the browned patties on the baking sheet and bake until completely cooked through, about 15 minutes.

7. Serve on the lettuce leaves, topped with the avocado slices.

Nutrition:

Calories: 374

Fat: 33g

Protein: 18g

Carbohydrates: 3g

Fiber: 2g

52

Herb Butter Scallops

Preparation Time: 10 minutes
Cooking Time: 10 minutes
Servings: 3
Ingredients:

- 1 pound sea scallops, cleaned
- Freshly ground black pepper
- 8 tablespoons butter, divided
- 2 teaspoons minced garlic
- Juice of 1 lemon
- 2 teaspoons chopped fresh basil
- 1 teaspoon chopped fresh thyme

Directions:

1. Pat the scallops dry with paper towels and season them lightly with pepper.
2. Place a large skillet over medium heat and add 2 tablespoons of butter.
3. Arrange the scallops in the skillet, evenly spaced but not too close together, and sear each side until they are golden brown, about 2½ minutes per side.
4. Remove the scallops to a plate and set aside.

5. Add the remaining 6 tablespoons of butter to the skillet and sauté the garlic until translucent, about 3 minutes.
6. Stir in the lemon juice, basil, and thyme and return the scallops to the skillet, turning to coat them in the sauce.
7. Serve immediately.

Nutrition:
Calories: 306
Fat: 24g
Protein: 19g
Carbohydrates: 4g
Fiber: 0g

53

Paprika Chicken

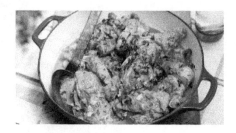

Preparation Time: 10 minutes
Cooking Time: 25 minutes
Servings: 4
Ingredients:

- 4 (4-ounce) chicken breasts, skin-on
- Sea salt
- Freshly ground black pepper
- 1 tablespoon olive oil
- ½ cup chopped sweet onion
- ½ cup heavy (whipping) cream
- 2 teaspoons smoked paprika
- ½ cup sour cream
- 2 tablespoons chopped fresh parsley

Directions:

1. Lightly season the chicken with salt and pepper.

2. Place a large skillet over medium-high heat and add the olive oil.
3. Sear the chicken on both sides until almost cooked through, about 15 minutes in total. Remove the chicken to a plate.
4. Add the onion to the skillet and sauté until tender, about 4 minutes.
5. Stir in the cream and paprika and bring the liquid to a simmer.
6. Return the chicken and any accumulated juices to the skillet and simmer the chicken for 5 minutes until completely cooked.
7. Stir in the sour cream and remove the skillet from the heat.
8. Serve topped with the parsley.

Nutrition:
Calories: 389
Fat: 30g
Protein: 25g
Carbohydrates: 4g
Fiber: 0g

54

Trout and Chili Nuts

Preparation Time: 10 minutes
Cooking time: 0 minutes
Servings: 3
Ingredients:

- 1.5kg of rainbow trout
- 300gr shelled walnuts
- 1 bunch of parsley
- 9 cloves of garlic
- 7 tablespoons of olive oil
- 2 fresh hot peppers
- The juice of 2 lemons
- Halls

Directions:

1. Clean and dry the trout then place them in a baking tray.
2. Chop the walnuts, parsley and chili peppers then mash the garlic cloves.
3. Mix the ingredients by adding olive oil, lemon juice and a pinch of salt.
4. Stuff the trout with some of the sauce and use the rest to cover the fish.
5. Bake at 180° for 30/40 minutes.

6. Serve the trout hot or cold.

Nutrition:

Calories 226

Fat 5

Fiber 2

Carbs 7

Protein 8

55

Nut Granola & Smoothie Bowl

Preparation Time: 10 minutes
Cooking time: 40 minutes
Servings: 3
Ingredients:

- 6 cups Greek yogurt
- 4 tablespoon almond butter
- A handful toasted walnuts
- 3 tablespoon unsweetened cocoa powder
- 4 teaspoon swerve brown sugar
- 2 cups nut granola for topping

Directions:

1. Combine the Greek yogurt, almond butter, walnuts, cocoa powder, and swerve brown sugar in a smoothie maker; puree in high-speed until smooth and well mixed.
2. Share the smoothie into four breakfast bowls, top with a half cup of granola each, and serve.

Nutrition:
Kcal 361,
Fat 31.2g,
Net Carbs 2g,

Protein 13g

56

Bacon and Egg Quesadillas

Preparation Time: 10 minutes
Cooking time: 30 minutes
Servings: 3
Ingredients:

- 8 low carb tortilla shells
- 6 eggs
- 1 cup water
- 3 tablespoon butter
- 1 ½ cups grated cheddar cheese
- 1 ½ cups grated Swiss cheese
- 5 bacon slices
- 1 medium onion, thinly sliced
- 1 tablespoon chopped parsley

Directions

1. Bring the eggs to a boil in water over medium heat for 10 minutes. Transfer the eggs to an ice water bath, peel the shells, and chop them; set aside.
2. Meanwhile, as the eggs cook, fry the bacon in a skillet over medium heat for 4 minutes until crispy. Remove and chop. Plate and set aside too.

3. Fetch out 2/3 of the bacon fat and sauté the onions in the remaining grease over medium heat for 2 minutes; set aside. Melt 1 tablespoon of butter in a skillet over medium heat.
4. Lay one tortilla in a skillet; sprinkle with some Swiss cheese. Add some chopped eggs and bacon over the cheese, top with onion, and sprinkle with some cheddar cheese. Cover with another tortilla shell. Cook for 45 seconds, then carefully flip the quesadilla, and cook the other side too for 45 seconds. Remove to a plate and repeat the cooking process using the remaining tortilla shells.
5. Garnish with parsley and serve warm.

Nutrition:
Kcal 449,
Fat 48.7g,
Net Carbs 6.8g,
Protein 29.1g

57

Bacon and Cheese Frittata

Preparation Time: 10 minutes
Cooking time: 20 minutes
Servings: 3
Ingredients:

* 10 slices bacon
* 10 fresh eggs
* 3 tablespoon butter, melted
* ½ cup almond milk
* Salt and black pepper to taste
* 1 ½ cups cheddar cheese, shredded
* ¼ cup chopped green onions

Directions:

1. Preheat the oven to 400ºF and grease a baking dish with cooking spray. Cook the bacon in a skillet over medium heat for 6 minutes. Once crispy, remove from the skillet to paper towels and discard grease. Chop into small pieces. Whisk the eggs, butter, milk, salt, and black pepper. Mix in the bacon and pour the mixture into the baking dish.
2. Sprinkle with cheddar cheese and green onions, and bake in the oven for 10 minutes or until the eggs are thoroughly cooked. Re-

move and cool the frittata for 3 minutes, slice into wedges, and serve warm with a dollop of Greek yogurt.

Nutrition:
Kcal 325,
Fat 28g,
Net Carbs 2g,
Protein 15g

58

Spicy Egg Muffins with Bacon & Cheese

Preparation Time: 10 minutes
Cooking time: 20 minutes
Servings: 3
Ingredients:

- 12 eggs
- ¼ cup coconut milk
- Salt and black pepper to taste
- 1 cup grated cheddar cheese
- 12 slices bacon
- 4 jalapeño peppers, seeded and minced

Directions:

1. Preheat oven to 370ºF.
2. Crack the eggs into a bowl and whisk with coconut milk until combined. Season with salt and pepper, and evenly stir in the cheddar cheese.
3. Line each hole of a muffin tin with a slice of bacon and fill each with the egg mixture two-thirds way up. Top with the jalapeno peppers and bake in the oven for 18 to 20 minutes or until puffed and golden. Remove, allow cooling for a few minutes, and serve with arugula salad.

Nutrition:
Kcal 302,
Fat 23.7g,
Net Carbs 3.2g,
Protein 20g

59

Ham & Egg Broccoli Bake

Preparation Time: 10 minutes
Cooking time: 25 minutes
Servings: 3
Ingredients:

- 2 heads broccoli, cut into small florets
- 2 red bell peppers, seeded and chopped
- ¼ cup chopped ham
- 2 teaspoon ghee
- 1 teaspoon dried oregano + extra to garnish
- Salt and black pepper to taste
- 8 fresh eggs

Directions

1. Preheat oven to 425ºF.
2. Melt the ghee in a frying pan over medium heat; brown the ham, stirring frequently, about 3 minutes.
3. Arrange the broccoli, bell peppers, and ham on a foil-lined baking sheet in a single layer, toss to combine; season with salt, oregano, and black pepper. Bake for 10 minutes until the vegetables have softened.

4. Remove, create eight indentations with a spoon, and crack an egg into each. Return to the oven and continue to bake for an additional 5 to 7 minutes until the egg whites are firm.
5. Season with salt, black pepper, and extra oregano, share the bake into four plates and serve with strawberry lemonade (optional).

Nutrition:
Kcal 344,
Fat 28g,
Net Carbs 4.2g,
Protein 11g

60

Hot Buffalo wings

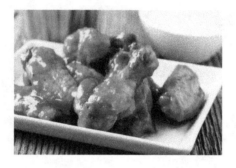

Preparation Time: 10 minutes
Cooking Time: 47 minutes
Servings: 3
Ingredients:

- Hot sauce ¼ cup
- Coconut oil 4 tablespoons, plus more for rubbing on the wings
- Chicken wings 12 (fresh or frozen)
- Garlic 1 clove, minced
- Salt ¼ teaspoon
- Paprika ¼ teaspoon
- Cayenne pepper ¼ teaspoon
- Ground black pepper 1 dash

Directions:

1. Preheat your oven to 400 degrees F (200 degrees C).
2. Evenly spread chicken wings on a wire rack placed on a baking dish (it will save wings to become soggy on the bottom).
3. Rub each chicken wing with olive oil and season with salt and pepper, then bake for 45 minutes, or until crispy.
4. Meanwhile, in a saucepan combine coconut oil and garlic and cook over medium heat for 1 minute, or until fragrant.
5. Remove from heat and stir in hot sauce, salt, paprika, cayenne pepper and black pepper.
6. Remove wings from the oven and transfer to a large bowl.
7. Pour hot sauce mixture over wings and toss until each wing is coated with the sauce.
8. Serve immediately.

Nutrition:
Calories: 391
Carbohydrates: 1 g
Fats: 33 g
Protein: 31 g

61

Turkey Meatballs

Preparation Time: 30 minutes
Cooking Time: 0 minutes
Servings: 4
Ingredients:

- 255g turkey sausage
- 2 tablespoons of extra virgin olive oil
- One can of 425g chickpeas, rinsed and drained...
- 1/2 medium onion, chopped, 2/3 cup
- 2 cloves of garlic, finely chopped
- 1 teaspoon of cumin
- 1/2 cup flour
- 1/2 teaspoon instant yeast for desserts
- Salt and ground black pepper
- 1 cup of Greek yogurt
- 2 tablespoons of lime juice
- 2 radicchio hearts, chopped
- Hot sauce

Directions:

1. Preheat the oven to 200°C.
2. In a processor, blend the chickpeas, onion, garlic, cumin, 1 teaspoon salt and 1/2 teaspoon pepper until all the ingredients are

finely chopped. Add the flour, baking powder and blend to make everything mix well. Transfer to a medium bowl and add the sausage, stirring together with your hands. Cover and refrigerate for 30 minutes.

3. Once cold, take the mixture in spoonful, forming 1-inch balls with wet hands. Heat the olive oil in a pan over medium heat. In two groups, put the falafel in the pan and cook until slightly brown, about a minute and a half per side. Transfer to a baking tray and bake in the oven until well cooked, for about 10 minutes.

4. Mix together the yogurt, lime juice, 1/2 teaspoon salt and 1/4 teaspoon pepper. Divide the lettuce into 4 plates, season with some yogurt sauce.

Nutrition:

Calories 189

Fat 5

Protein 77

Sugar 3

62

Chicken in Sweet and Sour Sauce with Corn Salad

Preparation Time: 10 minutes
Cooking Time: 15 minutes
Servings: 4
Ingredients:

- 2 cups plus 2 tablespoons of unflavored low-fat yoghurt
- 2 cups of frozen mango chunks
- 3 tablespoons of honey
- ¼ cup plus 1 tablespoon apple cider vinegar
- ¼ cup sultana
- 2 tablespoons of olive oil, plus an amount to be brushed
- ¼ teaspoon of cayenne pepper
- 5 dried tomatoes (not in oil)
- 2 small cloves of garlic, finely chopped
- 4 cobs, peeled
- 8 peeled and boned chicken legs, peeled (about 700g)
- Halls
- 6 cups of mixed salad
- 2 medium carrots, finely sliced

Directions:

1. For the smoothie: in a blender, mix 2 cups of yogurt, 2 cups of ice, 1 cup of mango and all the honey until the mixture becomes completely smooth. Divide into 4 glasses and refrigerate until ready to use. Rinse the blender.
2. Preheat the grill to medium-high heat. Mix the remaining cup of mango, ¼ cup water, ¼ cup vinegar, sultanas, olive oil, cayenne pepper, tomatoes and garlic in a microwave bowl. Cover with a piece of clear film and cook in the microwave until the tomatoes become soft, for about 3 minutes. Leave to cool slightly and pass in a blender. Transfer to a small bowl. Leave 2 tablespoons aside to garnish, turn the chicken into the remaining mixture.
3. Put the corn on the grill, cover and bake, turning it over if necessary, until it is burnt, about 10 minutes. Remove and keep warm.
4. Brush the grill over medium heat and brush the grills with a little oil. Turn the chicken legs into half the remaining sauce and ½ teaspoon of salt. Put on the grill and cook until the cooking marks appear and the internal temperature reaches 75°C on an instantaneous thermometer, 8 to 10 minutes per side. Bart and sprinkle a few times with the remaining sauce while cooking.
5. While the chicken is cooking, beat the remaining 2 tablespoons of yogurt, the 2 tablespoons of sauce set aside, the remaining spoonful of vinegar, 1 tablespoon of water and ¼ teaspoon of salt in a large bowl. Mix the mixed salad with the carrots. Divide chicken, corn and salad into 4 serving dishes. Garnish the salad with the dressing set aside. Serve each plate with a mango smoothie.

Nutrition:
Calories 346
Protein 56
Fat 45

63

Chinese Chicken Salad

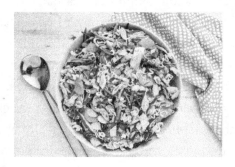

Preparation Time: 15 minutes
Cooking Time: 30 minutes
Servings: 4
Ingredients:

- For the chicken salad:
- 4 divided chicken breasts with skin and bones
- Olive oil of excellent quality
- Salt and freshly ground black pepper
- 500 g asparagus, with the ends removed and cut into three parts diagonally
- 1 red pepper, peeled
- Chinese condiment, recipe to follow
- 2 spring onions (both the white and the green part), sliced diagonally
- 1 tablespoon of white sesame seeds, toasted

- For Chinese dressing:
- 120 ml vegetable oil
- 60 ml of apple cider vinegar of excellent quality
- 60 ml soy sauce
- 1 ½ tablespoon of black sesame
- ½ tablespoon of honey
- 1 clove of garlic, minced
- ½ teaspoon of fresh peeled and grated ginger
- ½ tablespoon sesame seeds, toasted
- 60 g peanut butter
- 2 teaspoons of salt
- ½ teaspoons freshly ground black pepper

Directions:

1. For the chicken salad:
2. Heat the oven to 180°C (or 200°C for gas oven). Put the chicken breast on a baking tray and rub the skin with a little olive oil. Season freely with salt and pepper.
3. Brown for 35 to 40 minutes, until the chicken is freshly cooked. Let it cool down as long as it takes to handle it. Remove the meat from the bones, remove the skin and chop the chicken into medium-sized pieces.
4. Blanch the asparagus in a pot of salted water for 3-5 minutes until tender. Soak them in water with ice to stop cooking. Drain them. Cut the peppers into strips the same size as the asparagus. In a large bowl, mix the chopped chicken, asparagus and peppers.
5. Spread the Chinese dressing on chicken and vegetables. Add the spring onions and sesame seeds, and season to taste. Serve cold or at room temperature.
6. For Chinese dressing:
7. Mix all ingredients and set aside until use.

Nutrition:
Calories 222
Protein 28
Fat 10
Sugar 6

64

Chicken Salad

Preparation Time: 15 minutes
Cooking Time: 25 minutes
Servings: 4
Ingredients:

- For the Buffalo chicken salad:
- 2 chicken breasts (225 g) peeled, boned, cut in half
- 2 tablespoons of hot cayenne pepper sauce (or another type of hot sauce), plus an addition depending on taste
- 2 tablespoons of olive oil
- 2 romaine lettuce heart, cut into 2 cm strips
- 4 celery stalks, finely sliced
- 2 carrots, roughly grated
- 2 fresh onions, only the green part, sliced
- 125 ml of blue cheese dressing, recipe to follow
- For the seasoning of blue cheese
- 2 tablespoons mayonnaise
- 70 ml of partially skimmed buttermilk
- 70 ml low-fat white yoghurt
- 1 tablespoon of wine vinegar
- ½ teaspoon of sugar
- 35 g of chopped blue cheese
- Salt and freshly ground black pepper

Directions:

1. For the Buffalo chicken salad:
2. Preheat the grid.
3. Place the chicken between 2 sheets of baking paper and beat it with a meat tenderizer so that it is about 2 cm thick, then cut the chicken sideways creating 1 cm strips.
4. In a large bowl, add the hot sauce and oil, add the chicken and turn it over until it is well soaked. Place the chicken on a baking tray and grill until well cooked, about 4-6 minutes, turning it once.
5. In a large bowl, add the lettuce, celery, grated carrots and fresh onions. Add the seasoning of blue cheese. Distribute the vegetables in 4 plates and arrange the chicken on each of the dishes. Serve with hot sauce on the side.
6. For the blue cheese dressing:
7. Cover a small bowl with absorbent paper folded in four. Spread the yoghurt on the paper and put it in the fridge for 20 minutes to drain and firm it.
8. In a medium bowl, beat the buttermilk and firm yogurt with mayonnaise until well blended. Add the vinegar and sugar and keep beating until well blended. Add the blue cheese and season with salt and pepper to taste.

Nutrition:
321 calories
Fat 3
Fiber 5
Carbs 7
Protein 4

65

Avocado and Kale Eggs

Preparation Time: 10 minutes
Cooking time: 30 minutes
Servings: 3
Ingredients:

- 1 teaspoon ghee
- 1 red onion, sliced
- 4 oz. chorizo, sliced into thin rounds
- 1 cup chopped kale
- 1 ripe avocado, pitted, peeled, chopped
- 4 eggs
- Salt and black pepper to season

Directions:

1. Preheat oven to 370ºF.
2. Melt ghee in a cast iron pan over medium heat and sauté the onion for 2 minutes. Add the chorizo and cook for 2 minutes more, flipping once.
3. Introduce the kale in batches with a splash of water to wilt, season lightly with salt, stir and cook for 3 minutes. Mix in the avocado and turn the heat off.
4. Create four holes in the mixture, crack the eggs into each hole, sprinkle with salt and black pepper, and slide the pan into the pre-

heated oven to bake for 6 minutes until the egg whites are set or firm and yolks still runny. Season to taste with salt and pepper, and serve right away with low carb toasts.

Nutrition:
Kcal 274,
Fat 23g,
Net Carbs 4g,
Protein 13g

66

Tofu Meat and Salad

Preparation Time: 15 minutes
Cooking Time: 20 minutes
Servings: 3
Ingredients:

- 1 tablespoon of garlic sauce and chili in a bottle
- 1 1/2 tablespoon sesame oil
- 3 tablespoons of low-sodium soy sauce
- 60 ml hoisin sauce
- 2 tablespoons rice vinegar
- 2 tablespoons of sherry or Chinese cooking wine
- 225 g of extra-solid tofu
- 2 teaspoons of rapeseed oil
- 2 tablespoons of finely chopped fresh ginger
- 4 spring onions, with the green part chopped and set aside, in thin slices
- 225 g of minced lean beef (90% or more lean)
- 25 g of diced Chinese water chestnuts
- 1 large head of cappuccino lettuce, with the leaves separated, but without the outer ones
- 1 red pepper, diced

Directions:

- In a bowl, mix together the garlic and chili sauce, sesame oil, soy sauce, hoisin sauce, vinegar and sherry.
- Cut the tofu into 1 cm thick slices and place them on a kitchen towel. Use the cloth to dab the tofu well to remove as much water as possible. Should take a couple of minutes and about three dish towels. Chop the dry tofu well and set aside.
- Heat the oil in a wok or in a very large pan and medium flame. Add the ginger and the white part of the spring onions and cook until the spring onions become translucent and the ginger fragrant, for about 2-3 minutes. Add the beef and tofu and cook, stirring, until the meat becomes dull and freshly cooked, for about 4-5 minutes. Add the sauce set aside. Reduce the flame and simmer slowly, stirring, for another 3-4 minutes. Add the chestnuts and mix well to incorporate.
- Fill each lettuce leaf with stuffing. Serve by decorating with the green part of the spring onions, red pepper and peanuts.

Nutrition:
Calories 122
Fat 2
Protein 66

67

Asparagus and Pistachios Vinaigrette

Preparation Time: 10 minutes
Cooking Time: 5minutes
Servings: 2
Ingredients:

- Two 455g bunches of large asparagus, without the tip
- 1 tablespoon of olive oil
- Salt and freshly ground black pepper
- 6 tablespoons of sliced pistachios blanched and boiled
- 1 1/2 tablespoon lemon juice
- 1/4 teaspoon of sugar
- 1 1/2 teaspoon lemon zest

Directions:

1. Preheat the oven to 220°C. Put the grill in the top third of the oven. Place the asparagus on a baking tray covered with baking paper. Sprinkle with olive oil and season with a little salt and pepper. Bake for 15 minutes, until soft.
2. Meanwhile, blend 5 tablespoons of almonds, lemon juice, sugar and 6 tablespoons of water for 1 minute until smooth. Taste and regulate salt. Pour the sauce on a plate and put the spinach on the sauce. Decorate with peel and the remaining spoon of pistachios

Nutrition:
Calories 560
Fat 5
Fiber 2
Carbs 3
Protein 9